# OPPORTUNISTIC INFECTIONS
# IN CANCER PATIENTS

# OPPORTUNISTIC INFECTIONS IN CANCER PATIENTS

**J. Aubertin and J. Y. Lacut**
Infectious Diseases Clinic
University of Bordeaux II, France

**B. Hoerni and M. Durand**
Bergonie Foundation
University of Bordeaux II, France

Translation from the original French edition adapted by

## DONALD ARMSTRONG, M.D., F.A.C.P.

Chief, Infectious Disease Service
Memorial Sloan-Kettering Cancer Center
New York, New York
Director of the Microbiology Laboratory
Memorial Sloan-Kettering Cancer Center
Professor of Medicine
Cornell University Medical College
New York, New York

MASSON    Publishing    USA,    Inc.
New York • Paris • Barcelona • Milan

Original French Edition:

*LES INFECTIONS CHEZ LES CANCEREUX*

by J. Aubertin, J. Y. Lacut, B. Hoerni, and M. Durand, 1976.

ISBN 0-89352-014-4

Library of Congress Catalog Number: 77-94828

Printed in the United States of America

# Preface

Infections are the most common single cause of death in patients with neoplastic disease. If their infections are anticipated, preventive, diagnostic, and therapeutic measures can be highly effective. Anticipation requires knowledge of the factors that make a patient susceptible to various types of infections with specific microorganisms. A person with Hodgkin's disease who develops menigitis caused by *Listeria monocytogenes* is immunosuppressed in a different manner than the individual with acute leukemia who develops *Pseudomonas aeruginosa* bacteremia from ulcers in the gastrointestinal tract. Knowledge of the immune defects caused by the underlying disease plus alterations caused by therapy is necessary for understanding the pathogenesis of infections in immunosuppressed patients and for directing approaches toward control and treatment. The authors have attempted to set the stage and direct the clinician in evaluating such patients.

Although I do not agree with their conclusions in some instances, I do believe that it is important to attempt to bring together the factors that make patients with neoplastic disease more susceptible to infection and to try to anticipate the infection by knowing the clinical setting in which they occur and the best methods for rapid diagnosis and treatment. Preventive measures including vaccination and/or hyperimmune globulin against prevalent organisms plus granulocylte transfusions should become more important as we develop better methods of using them effectively.

Finally, the best method of preventing infections in neoplastic disease is to effectively treat the neoplasm, and likewise an essential part of treating established infection is to induce a remission of the neoplasm.

Donald Armstrong, M.D.

# Introduction

Ten years ago, infections in cancer patients attracted little attention. The common suppuration of ulcerated cancers, the frequency of herpes zoster in all cancers, as well as infections of any kind in Hodgkin's patients were all well recognized. Nevertheless, the descriptions of infections were rare, and either by the nature of the responsible etiological agent or by the cancer involved, had just begun.

Today, infection and cancer are considered as old friends (DeVita and Young, 1973), but the binds which link them together are now seen from a new point of view. This change is the result of increasing attention given to infection, which has lead to a better understanding of its actual importance and place in cancer patients and is due, even more, to a transformation of pathology. This evolution depends on modifications in microbial ecology and renewal of infectious pathology (Gaya *et al.*, 1973). It also depends on the progress of anticancer therapy: since these patients are living longer, it is not surprising that they develop superinfections; at the same time, the anticancer treatment impairs host defense mechanisms, favoring infectious complications. Thus, cancer and infections are closely related and anticancer therapy plays an intermediary role.

Many cancers cannot be treated successfully without aggressive chemotherapy and thus without important toxicity and infectious risks for the patient. Hence management of these infections becomes essential for the continuation and efficacious improvement of anticancer treatment. For example, in acute leukemias, especially the myeloid form, the results obtained depend on the anti-infectious means of each cancer center (O.E.R.T.C., 1975).

Oncologists are directly concerned with cancer–infection problems as the quality of patient survival is related to them. Infectious disease specialists are also concerned as they are confronted with new aspects of infectious pathology owing to the responsible microorganisms as well as to the clinical aspect of the infection. Moreover, these particular infections are also observed in other patients suffering immunosuppression.

These problems have been particularly studied in all important oncology centers, in the United States in New York at the Memorial Sloan-Kettering Cancer Center with D. Armstrong; in Houston at the M. D. Anderson Hospital with G. P. Bodey and V. Rodriguez; in Maryland at the NCI with A. S. Levine and S. S. Schimpff and in Europe in Brussels at the Jules-Bordet Institute with J. Klastersky; in London, at the Hammersmith Hospital with H. Gaya and H. N. Tattersall; in Paris in the Hematology Services of J. Bernard, J. Bousser, B. Dreyfus, and G. Mathé.

In Bordeaux, over the past years, we have organized a medical team joining oncologists and infectious disease specialists. We have mainly oriented our studies toward current problems which concern cancer patients in general, but without omitting rarer pathology which we have had the opportunity to observe.

We wish to express our appreciation to Professor Cl. Lagarde, Director of the Bergonié Foundation, for his invaluable aid and extend our thanks to our colleagues for their technical help and constructive criticisms, particularly Dr. Jacques Chauvergne, Head of the Department of Internal Medicine, and Dr. Geneviève Hoerni-Simon, Head of the Hematology Division of the Bergonié Foundation. Our work has been greatly assisted by the Laboratory of Microbiology headed by Prof. Ag. J. Latrille, Chairman of The University of Bordeaux. Finally we wish to acknowledge Dr. C. Tancrède, Head of the Clinical Microbiology Department of the Gustave-Roussy Institute at Villejuif for his very excellent criticism.

# Contents

Preface by Donald Armstrong, M.D.                                      iii

Introduction                                                            v

**Part 1. Fundamentals**

1. Epidemiology                                                         3
     Frequency of Infections in Cancer Patients                        4
     Importance of Cancers at the Origin of
       Certain Infections                                             11
     Importance of Infections at the Origin of
       Certain Manifestations in Cancer Patients                      13
     Epidemiologic Problems                                           14
2. Factors Favoring Infections in Cancer Patients                     16
     Predisposing Factors                                             16
     Tumor                                                            18
     Medical Intervention                                             22
3. Pathophysiology                                                    29
     Microbial Contamination                                          29
     From Contamination to Infection                                  31
     Patient–Cancer–Infection Relationship                            32
     Fever in Cancer Patients                                         37
4. General Diagnostic Problems                                        42
     Clinical Diagnosis                                               42
     Biologic Diagnosis                                               53

**Part 2. Diagnosis and Clinical Manifestations**

5. Bacterial Infections                                               65
     Localized Infections                                             66
     Septicemias                                                      72
     Mycobacterial Infections                                         85
6. Viral Infections                                                   90
     Herpes zoster and Varicella                                      92
     Other Infections Caused by Herpes Virus                          99
     Other Viral Infections                                          101

7.  Fungal Infections                                      103
        General Information                                103
        Candidiasis                                        106
        Aspergillosis                                      109
        Other Fungal Infections                            113
8.  Parasitic Infections                                   116
        Toxoplasmosis                                      116
        Pneumocystosis                                     120
        Other Parasitosis                                  125

**Part 3. Treatment and Evolution**

9.  Preventive Treatments                                  129
        Anticancer Treatment                               129
        Anti-Infectious Treatments                         132
10. Curative Treatment                                     140
        Anti-Infectious Chemotherapy                       140
        Nonspecific Treatment                              150
11. Evolution and Prognosis                                154
        Interlocking Pathology                             155
        Lethal Infections                                  157
        Prognosis of Infected Cancer Patients              159
    Conclusion                                             161
    References                                             163
    Index                                                  193

# 1

# Fundamentals

# CHAPTER 1

# Epidemiology

All doctors are aware that infections are particularly frequent in Hodgkin's disease and, since the first paper of Dubin (1947), many publications have dealt with this problem. They are equally aware that herpes virus infections, particularly herpes zoster, are often observed in cancer patients. What remains to be done, however, is to state precisely the general importance and frequency of infections for all cancer patients. There are various ways to approach the subject, but often, as we shall see, they are not complete.

The increasing number of publications dealing with this problem probably has little to do with the increasing incidence of these infections during the past few years; rather it is due to the growing attention they receive especially because of their particular characteristics and the development of their control.

There are no important global statistics which cover all types of cancer. The published data need to be interpreted, as they may vary considerably depending on the observer's point of view (Table I). If hospitalization periods are alone considered, one favors the representation of severe infections. If the patient is continually followed throughout the course of his disease and his illness is constantly surveyed, one can find banal infections such as herpes zoster or "flus" that have not been thoroughly studied or diagnosed. If only terminal-stage infections are considered (verified by necropsies), one selects cancers with poor evolution. Other variations are due to the conditions of patient recruitment and the type of service which publishes the study. Different infections are observed in pediatric and in adult services, in infectious disease and oncology services, and for the latter, in its surgical and medical sections (more or less specialized in hematology).

It is not surprising, for example, that in an infectious disease service 40% of cancer patients suffer infections (Lacut *et al.*, 1974), whereas in an oncology service this percentage is only 21% (Durand *et al.*, 1974), although the distribution of diverse tumoral types is comparable in both series. In addition, a certain diversity, easier to detect, can be attributed to the geographic repartition of some infections.

Finally, to complete the list of factors which cause certain apparent variations, the diagnostic conditions must be considered. When diagnosis

3

TABLE I.   Characteristics of Infections According to the Origin of Patients

| | Origin | Infections |
|---|---|---|
| Inpatients | Cancer center | Representative infections but variable according to the Service: radiotherapy, surgery, medicine, etc. |
| | Infectious disease department | Severe or particular infections |
| | Hematology department | Infections particular to malignant blood diseases |
| | Children's hospital | Importance of malignant blood disease infections particular to children |
| | All hospitals | Variations according to geography and microbial ecology |
| Outpatients | | Census of mild infections |

is made prior to clinical manifestations, with the support of some complementary investigations, there is little room for discussion. On the contrary, it is often difficult to interpret serologic variations when serologic tests have been performed systematically without any clinical symptom of infection: these variations may be due to latent infection or to nonspecific reactions. The problem is the same when microorganisms are discovered at a necropsy: their discovery does not necessarily affirm their responsibility in a lethal infection, as their presence may only be due to premortem contamination.

The importance of diverse cancers as the source of principal infections shall be discussed in later chapters concerning each type of infection. In this chapter, we shall indicate the relative frequency of diverse infections which are at the cause of certain pathologic manifestations, along with other causes, particularly turmoral or therapeutic. Finally, the so-called epidemiologic variations shall be briefly considered. Throughout the entire chapter we shall try to take into consideration the aforementioned variable factors in an effort to allow an exact interpretation of the data.

## FREQUENCY OF INFECTIONS IN CANCER PATIENTS

### Global Statistics

For an overall view we shall cite the figures observed in a medical oncology service for a hospitalization period which, on the average, lasted 29 days and corresponded to 176 febrile infections for 1162 patients (Table II).

TABLE II.  Frequency of Infections in Hospitalized Cancer Patients[a]

| Site of the Cancers | Total Number of Patients | Number of Infections | Percentages |
|---|---|---|---|
| Bone marrow and lymph nodes | 314 | 29 | 9.2 |
| Breast | 194 | 32 | 16.5 |
| Uterus | 67 | 26 | 38.8 |
| Head and neck | 142 | 33 | 23.2 |
| Esophagus | 43 | 21 | 48.8 |
| Bronchi | 46 | 23 | 50.0 |
| Digestive tract | 87 | 4 | 4.6 |
| Skin | 67 | 4 | 6.0 |
| Miscellaneous | 202 | 4 | 1.9 |
| Total | 1162 | 176 | 15.1 |

[a] From Durand et al. (1974), 1972–1973; Cancer Center, Bordeaux, France.

In an investigation concerning all followed-up cancers in a cancer center we have noted, for an observation period of approximately 40 months per patient, that an anti-infectious treatment had been given to more than 50% of the patients. This treatment included simple local disinfection for 40% of the patients or general antibiotic treatment for 28% (Hoerni et al., 1976). The problems dealt with are often banal, but their extreme frequency in oncology gives them an indisputable importance. Table III gives the repartition of some infectious agents and Table IV gives the repartition of the perianal and perirectal infections in relation to the main types of cancer.

A dozen publications have been compiled and compared by Gaya et al. (1973), but for the most part, they concern only leukemic patients. Most of the publications deal either with a particular infection or with a particular cancer. First we will review the frequency of certain infections in cancer patients.

## Incidence of Certain Infections

**Bacterial Infections.** For 68,675 incoming patients enrolled at M.D. Anderson Hospital between 1960 and 1968, 33 cases of salmonellosis were observed [16 patients with hematologic malignancies (Sinkovics and Smith, 1969)].

For tuberculosis, the census of 210 cases observed in more than 50,000 cancer patients between 1950 and 1971 at Memorial Center demonstrated that the prevalence of this infection is highest among the respiratory cancers and malignant lymphomas (around 1%); intermediary for head and neck cancers, gastric tumors, and acute lymphoid leukemia

TABLE III.  Distribution of Infectious Agents According to the Type of Cancer[a]

| Infectious Agent | Cancer[b] | | | | | |
|---|---|---|---|---|---|---|
| | Acute Myeloid Leukemia | Acute Lymphoid Leukemia | Chronic Myeloid Leukemia | Malignant Lymphomas | Solid Tumors | Miscellaneous |
| *Pseudomonas* | 18 | 4 | 0 | 30 | 40 | 8 |
| *Listeria* | 0 | 11 | 0 | 75 | 7 | 7 |
| *Cytomegalovirus* | 5 | 0 | 10 | 60 | 20 | 5 |
| *Candida* | 13 | 13 | 2 | 30 | 40 | 2 |
| *Aspergillus* | 17 | 28 | 7 | 30 | 16 | 2 |
| *Mucor* | 42 | 19 | 0 | 35 | 0 | 4 |
| *Cryptococcus* | 0 | 3 | 0 | 72 | 9 | 16 |
| *Toxoplasma* | 0 | 0 | 14 | 79 | 7 | 0 |

a From Armstrong (1973), Infectious Disease Department, Memorial Center, New York, New York.
b Figures are percentages for each agent.

TABLE IV.  Incidence of Perianal and Perirectal Infections in Cancer Patients[a]

| Type of Cancer | Number of Patients | Number of Infected Patients | Percentages |
|---|---|---|---|
| Acute nonlymphoid leukemia | 69 | 19 | 27 |
| Acute lymphoid leukemia | 24 | 2 | 8 |
| Multiple myeloma | 16 | 1 | 6 |
| Malignant lymphoma | 259 | 2[b] | 0.8 |
| Cerebral tumor | 67 | 1 | 1.5 |
| Solid metastasic tumor | 146 | 0 | 0 |
| Total | 581 | 25 | 4.3 |

[a] From Schimpff et al. (1972), 1962–1972, Baltimore Cencer Center.
[b] With leukemic evolution.

(around 0.5%); low for breast, intestinal, and urogenital cancers (around 0.1%). For a similar number of cancer patients, 129 cases of tuberculosis had been observed during 1950–1959 and only 64 during 1960–1969, which corresponds to a decreasing incidence of tuberculosis in the general population. One may note that none of the 2131 patients of this series with malignant melanoma had this infection (Kaplan et al., 1974).

**Viral Infections.**  In a Scandinavian general hospital, the observation of 147 cases of herpes zoster in more than 55,000 hospitalized patients demonstrated that the frequency of this infection was 9% in Hodgkin's patients, 3% in leukemias, 0.5% in other cancers, and 2% in noncancer patients (Wright and Winer, 1961).

In a series of 523 hematologic malignancies, herpes zoster was observed in 5.7% of all patients, 10% of chronic lymphoid leukemias, 8% of chronic myeloid leukemias, 4.6% of Hodgkin's disease, and none in cases of acute leukemia (Heine, 1965).

The incidence of herpes virus skin infections given by the most recent series is indicated in Table V, which clearly shows their predilection for Hodgkin's disease; this predilection is higher in diseases of a mixed cellularity (Wilson et al., 1974) or of a lymphoid depletion type (Monfardini et al., 1973).

In a series of 5788 consecutive necropsies in cancer patients, the diagnosis of cytomegalic inclusions disease was confirmed in 19 cases by the presence of intranuclear inclusions (Rosen and Hajdu, 1971). In a short series of 27 leukemic children, this diagnosis was confirmed by serodiagnosis in 6 patients, but only 3 had symptoms of the disease (Sutton et al., 1971). In a larger series of acute leukemias, clinical manifestations were due to cytomegalovirus in about 5% of the patients (Bussel et al., 1975).

TABLE V.   Incidence of Herpes Virus Skin Infections

| References | Types of Cancers[a] | | | |
| | Malignant Lymphomas | | | |
| | Hodgkin's Disease | Non-Hodgkin's Lymphomas | Leukemias | Solid Tumors |
| --- | --- | --- | --- | --- |
| Goffinet et al., 1972 | 15.4 | | | |
| Schimpff et al., 1972 | 25 | 8.7 | 2 | 1.8 |
| Wilson et al., 1974 | 19 | | | |
| Feldman et al., 1977[b] | 21.6 | | | |
| Monfardini et al., 1973 | 17 | 9 | | |
| Durand et al., 1976 | 20 | 8.5 | 3.9 | 4.9 |

[a] Figures are percentage of patients with infection.
[b] Children only.

**Fungal Infections.**   For 450 patients who died of hematologic malignancies from 1965 to 1971, 354 (79%) died of infections; among the 462 infectious episodes noted in these 354 patients, 31% were fungal infections (Levine et al., 1972). In a smaller series of 65 leukemic necropsies an analogous proportion (28%) of mycoses was observed (Mirsky and Cuttner, 1972). Systematic buccal cultures from 101 patients irradiated for head and neck cancers demonstrated that 30% were colonized by *Candida* before treatment; for the patients having negative cultures at the onset (Chen and Webster, 1974), one-half became positive during the irradiation.

*Torulopsis glabrata* was isolated 27 times in a series of 957 cancer patients observed between 1970 and 1974 (Aisner et al., 1976); in 17 patients there were clinical infectious symptoms, whereas in the 10 others the fungus was discovered only by routine necropsy (Table VI).

TABLE VI.   Incidence of *Torulopsis Glabrata* Infections in Cancer Patients[a]

| Type of Cancer | Total Number of Patients | Number of Checked Patients | Number of Infections |
| --- | --- | --- | --- |
| Solid tumor | 227 | 40 | 12 |
| Brain tumor | 115 | 17 | 2 |
| Malignant lymphoma | 398 | 48 | 6 |
| Myeloma | 17 | 4 | 0 |
| Acute leukemia | 158 | 52 | 7 |
| Chronic leukemia | 42 | 6 | 0 |
| Total | 957 | 167 | 27 |

[a] From Aisner et al. (1976), 1970–1974; Baltimore Cancer Center.

**Parasitic Infections.** The necropsies of 267 children with cancer, between 1954 and 1969 at M.D. Anderson Hospital in Houston, showed 15 cases of pneumocystosis, 9 of which were in leukemic patients [5% (Sedaghatian and Singer, 1972)]. Table VII gives the distribution of a larger series of pneumocystosis.

### Infectious Complications of Certain Cancers

Other series give the frequency of infections for a particular type of cancer.

Malignant blood diseases, and especially Hodgkin's disease, have been particularly studied for infectious complications. Table VIII juxtaposes the figures given by two series, one retaining only deceased and necropsied patients (Casazza et al., 1966), the other concerning all patients (Hoerni et al., 1971). Table VIII shows variations which depend on the selection of the patients. Another series of malignant lymphomas is given in Table IX. For the same period of observation, infections are three times more frequent for Hodgkin's lymphomas than for non-Hodgkin's lymphomas.

In a series of 100 children with acute lymphoid leukemia, all having been treated by an induction regimen consisting of vincristine and prednisone, one or several confirmed infectious episodes were observed in 51 cases and 19 patients had fever without an apparent infection. The remaining 30 children did not present any particular manifestation (Hughes and Smith, 1973).

In comparison with a control group of patients suffering from arteriosclerosis, patients with multiple myeloma experienced 15 times more infections, and those with chronic lymphoid leukemia five times more; half of these infections were pleuropulmonary and were linked to Gram-negative bacilli (Twomey, 1973). Chronic lymphoid leukemia predisposes much more to bacterial than to viral infections. Complicating infections appear to be especially frequent in hairy-cell leukemia: they herald the disease in one patient out of five and they constitute the main cause of death (Flandrin et al., 1973). Infections are also a frequent cause of death in patients with mycosis fungoides: they have been noted as the main cause of death in 40 out of 75 deceased patients (Epstein et al., 1972).

Infections are particularly frequent in ulcerated tumors of body cavities (upper respiratory tract, bronchi, gastrointestinal tract, and urogenital tract), but the analysis of their bacterial flora is very difficult, and thus no precise data regarding them can be found.

In Chapter 2 we shall indicate the frequency of infections for certain tumors after surgery.

TABLE VII.  Frequency of Pneumocystosis in Pediatric Cancers[a]

| Type of Cancer | Number of Patients | Number of Clinical Infections | Number of Occult Infections | Total Number of Infections |
|---|---|---|---|---|
| Acute lymphoid leukemia | 373 | 14 (3.7%) | 27 (7.3%) | 41 (11.0%) |
| Acute nonlymphoid leukemia | 100 | 0 | 8 | 8 |
| Malignant lymphoma | 62 | 3 | 1 | 4 |
| Neuroblastoma | 58 | 2 | 1 | 3 |
| Other solid tumors | 234 | 0 | 2 | 2 |
| Total | 827 | 19 (2.3%) | 39 (4.7%) | 58 (7.0%) |

[a] From Perera et al. (1970), 1962–1969, St. Jude Children's Hospital, Memphis, Tennessee.

TABLE VIII.   Frequency of Infections in Hodgkin's Disease

| | Casazza et al. (1966) | | Hoerni et al. (1971) | |
|---|---|---|---|---|
| Total number of patients | 51 | | 140 | |
| Bacterial infections | 56 | | 54 | |
| Septicemias | | 29 | | 6 |
| Bronchopulmonary system | | 14 | | 121 |
| Upper respiratory tract | | 0 | | 8 |
| Skin | | 4 | | 161 |
| Miscellaneous | | 9 | | 120 |
| Viral infections | 17 | | 53 | |
| Herpes zoster, varicella, herpes simplex | | 12 | | 27 |
| Others | | 5 | | 26 |
| Mycosis | 10 | | 8 | |
| Parasitic infections | 2 | | 8 | |
| Total | 85 | | 123 | |

TABLE IX.   Types of 411 Infections Observed in 629 Patients
with Malignant Lymphoma[a]

| | Infectious Agents | | | | | |
| Site | Bacteria | Virus | Fungus | Parasite | Undetermined | Total |
|---|---|---|---|---|---|---|
| Systemic | 26 | 7 | | 9 | 9 | 51 |
| Mouth and oropharynx | 10 | 12 | 18 | | | 40 |
| Respiratory tract | 74 | 38 | 2 | | 12 | 126 |
| Skin | 34 | 98 | 2 | | | 134 |
| Urogenital tract | 17 | | 2 | 2 | | 21 |
| Gastrointestinal tract | 8 | 7 | | 3 | | 18 |
| Meninges | 3 | | | | | 3 |
| Miscellaneous | 12 | 1 | 1 | 2 | 2 | 18 |
| Total | 184 | 163 | 25 | 16 | 23 | 411 |

[a] From Durand et al. (1975), 1960–1973, Cancer Center, Bordeaux, France.

## IMPORTANCE OF CANCERS AT THE ORIGIN
## OF CERTAIN INFECTIONS

Certain infections, the details of which will be discussed later, almost only develop when the host's defense is weakened (malnutrition, chronic illnesses, cancers, chemical immunosuppression, especially in organ transplanted patients). It is difficult to regroup figures concerning patients who have generally been dispersed in different hospital sections. There are, nevertheless, some publications which elucidate this subject.

In considering bacterial infections, it appears that malignant blood diseases predispose, above all, to septicemia and solid tumors predispose to pneumonia. The pneumonias are preponderant for cardiac transplants, the septicemias consequent to liver transplants, septicemias and pylonephritis following renal transplants, and patients who have received bone marrow grafts are candidates for all types of infections (Rodriguez et al., 1973).

Septicemias caused by *Staphylococcus albus* remain rare in cancer patients, whereas they are relatively frequent in patients with heart valve prothesis, cardiac pacemakers, or in drug addicts (Worms, 1969). For 20 cases of bacteremia caused by *Pseudomonas*, only 6 cancers (Iannini et al., 1974) were observed. For more than 300 infections caused by *Bacteroides*, cancer patients represented 27 cases, while the most frequent causes were related to surgical interventions for benign digestive or urogenital diseases (Okubadejo et al., 1973; Leigh, 1974).

In a series of 100 pneumonias caused by mycoplasmas, an underlying disease was found in 19 patients: sarcoidosis (8), systemic lupus (4), drepanocytosis (3), and Hodgkin's disease (4) (Putman et al., 1975).

For viral infections, 34 out of 147 cases of herpes zoster observed during hospitalization were linked to a cancer (Wright and Winer, 1961). In a series of 31 cases observed in children, 7 developed in cancer patients (Rogers and Tindall, 1972). Progressive multifocal leukoencephalopathy, linked to a papovavirus, is observed mainly in cancer patients, in particular, those with Hodgkin's disease or chronic lymphoid leukemia, but it is also observed during benign diseases which cause an immunodeficiency, such as sarcoidosis or certain types of tuberculosis (Escourolle et al., 1973).

For the mycosis, out of 13 cases of esophageal candidiasis, 5 appeared in leukemic patients, 4 in patients presenting bone marrow aplasia, and the 4 others in noncancer patients (Grève, 1964). The incidence is very different in the series of Moulinier et al. (1972) in which, out of 40 cases of esophageal candidiasis, 80% of them were secondary to a local (30%) or general (50%) cause, with only three cancer patients among them. Likewise in a series of 23 cases of abdominal candidiasis consisting of abscesses, infections of the cell wall, or fistulas, only four cancers and a majority of benign surgical illnesses (ulcers, bile tract diseases, appendicitis) were observed (Ackerman and Kronmueller, 1975).

In parasitic infections, out of 14 cases of pneumocystosis, 8 patients had cancers and 6 others were receiving corticosteroids (Forrest, 1972). In an American series (Leclair, 1969) of pneumocystosis, cancer was present in one-third of the cases along with premature births and children with congenital or malnutritive immunodeficiency, transplanted patients submitted to therapeutic immunosuppression, and a few patients with debilitating diseases such as systemic lupus. A large series grouping of nearly 200 cases of pneumocystosis demonstrated preexisting cancer in more than two-thirds of the patients (Table X). Out of 44 cases of severe

TABLE X.   Diseases Associated with Pneumocystosis[a]

|  | Number of Patients | Percentage |
|---|---|---|
| Cancers | 132 | 68.1 |
| Acute leukemia | 70 | 36.1 |
| Chronic leukemia | 21 | 10.8 |
| Hodgkin's disease | 21 | 10.8 |
| Non-Hodgkin's lymphoma | 13 | 6.7 |
| Solid tumor | 7 | 3.6 |
| Others | 62 | 31.9 |
| Primary immunodeficiency | 25 | 12.9 |
| Organ transplantation | 22 | 11.4 |
| Collagen disease | 9 | 4.6 |
| Miscellaneous | 6 | 3.1 |
| Total | 194 | 100 |

[a] From Walzer et al. (1974), 1967–1970, U.S.

anguillulosis, 11 developed in cancer patients; the others were in malnutrition cases, leprosy, or various chronically ill patients (Rivera et al., 1970; Purtillo et al., 1974).

## IMPORTANCE OF INFECTIONS AT THE ORIGIN OF CERTAIN MANIFESTATIONS IN CANCER PATIENTS

Certain pathologic manifestations of infections may cause the presenting signs or symptoms of cancer and may mainly create diagnostic problems which shall be discussed in detail in Chapter 4. Here we shall indicate a few figures which give the relative importance of the diverse causes at the origin of the most frequent manifestations.

Fever is the most important oncologic symptom, particularly for our purposes. Out of 526 recorded case histories in an infectious diseases service, 344 febrile episodes were noted and linked 146 times to neoplastic disease, 26 times to diverse causes (thrombophlebitis, lymphography, transfusion), while 26 times their origin could not be determined (Lacut et al., 1974). Fever, observed in 260 out of 1666 patients irradiated for cancer of the uterus, remained of unknown origin in more than one-half of the cases (57.3%), was linked to a pelvic inflammation—caused by cancer or irradiation—in 21.1% of the cases, to an infection in 11.1% of the patients, and to another cause in 10.4% (Van Herik, 1965).

Pulmonary manifestations are also frequent in cancer patients, but it is often difficult to determine their exact nature. A series of necropsies of 22 interstitial pneumopathies established a link between this illness and an infection in 16 cases (mainly pneumocystosis but also viral and mycotic infections), a metastasis in one case, a nonspecific illness in 2 cases, while in 3 cases the cause remained undetermined (Goodell et al., 1970). In 52 cases of pneumonia in patients with acute leukemia, a *Pseudomonas* was isolated 12 times, another bacterium 30 times, a *Candida* 12 times, and an *Aspergillus* 1 time (Sickles et al., 1973). In addition to lung cancers, pleuropulmonary radiologic changes are particularly frequent during leukemias, observed in 26% of the patients, mainly those with chronic lymphoid leukemia (41% of the cases); they are linked three times more often to an infection than to neoplastic disease (Voisin et al., 1970).

In one important series analyzing 795 neurologic manifestations observed in 5778 patients with malignant blood diseases, Williams et al. (1959) showed with precision that the peripheral nervous system, in addition to 118 spinal cord compressions and 202 involvements of peripheral or cranial nerves, there were 162 cases of herpes zoster. For the central nervous system, in addition to 112 cerebral metastases and 146 cerebromeningeal hemorrhages, there were 23 infections, the latter caused 10 times by a fungus, 8 times by a bacterium, 3 times by a virus, 1 time by toxoplasma, and 1 time by an undetermined agent.

Cutaneous manifestations are frequent in Hodgkin's disease: an early series indicated that 30% of the patients presented with pruritus, 20% with a neoplastic lesion, 20% with herpes zoster, and 10% with nonspecific lesions (Molander and Pack, 1968). In a more recent series of 94 patients, 4 presented with tumor involvement and 52 other cutaneous lesions, mainly pruritis (30) and herpes zoster (12), the other manifestations being paraneoplastic or intercurrent (Amblard et al., 1973).

## EPIDEMIOLOGIC PROBLEMS

Numerous variations can be noted from one country to another, from one hospital to another, and, for the same hospital service, from one period to another.

Geographical variations are especially apparent for microorganisms such as parasites and fungi, the majority of which appear much more frequently in North America than in Europe. The opposite is the case for toxoplasma, frequent in France and rare in the United States.

The hazards of "hospitalism" are well known. Here we shall only point out that the risk of pneumonia is estimated at 5% for hospitalized patients (Debusscher *et al.*, 1972). Attention has recently been given to the hazards caused by some fireproof material used for ceilings which harbors large quantities of different species of *Aspergillus* (Aisner *et al.*, 1976).

Variations in time intervals are also well known and should lead to a regular surveillance of the observed infections and the isolated micro-organisms in order to follow the microbial ecology of a hospital department. In a study on bacterial infections occurring during leukemia, Gaya *et al.* (1973), by their personal observations and those published elsewhere, found that the frequency of infections by *Pseudomonas* increased from 1959 to 1970, as did the group of *Klebsiella–Enterobacter*, while the frequency of *Staphylococcus aureus* remained constant or slightly diminished. For infections during multiple myeloma, those linked to *Pneumococcus*, which is classically the most frequent, have been outnumbered by Gram-negative infections, which represent three-quarters of the total in certain series (Meyers *et al.*, 1972). On the other hand, Tapper and Armstrong (1974) found that since 1971 the incidence of septicemia owing to *Pseudomonas* had diminished at Memorial Center.

These variations are largely due to medical evolution, particularly to the progress in treatments, anticancerous as well as anti-infectious, and they will be better understood by the end of Chapters 2 and 3, which describe the enhancing factors and the pathophysiology of infections in cancer patients.

# CHAPTER 2

# Factors Favoring Infections in Cancer Patients

As we have stated in Chapter 1, epidemiology shows that infections are more frequent in cancer patients than in the general population. Simple observation can explain that the frequency of contact caused by the multiplicity of disturbances found in cancer patients favors superinfection. First, we shall see that certain situations predispose to cancers as well as to infections. More often, the tumor is responsible for a particular susceptibility, local or general. Finally, medical interventions add factors which may have a decisive influence (Table XI).

## PREDISPOSING FACTORS

Certain patients present abnormalities, generalized or localized, congenital or acquired, which favor the development of an infection and the appearance of a cancer at the same time.

### Systemic Abnormalities

A rather rare but well-identified situation corresponds to immunologic deficiencies which facilitate, as one knows, the appearance of a cancer (Hoerni and Laporte, 1970; Kersey et al., 1973). Because of their preexisting deficiency, these patients are susceptible to infections and this susceptibility remains after the appearance of the neoplasm.

**Congenital Conditions.** The most frequent congenital condition is ataxia-telangiectasia, characterized by a deficiency of the cell-mediated immune response and an impaired synthesis of immunoglobulins (mainly the IgA) (Sedgwick and Boder, 1972). These patients frequently develop superinfections, particularly of the respiratory tract; they can coexist with a cancer which develops with a high frequency and most often involves the hematopoietic system (Hoerni et al., 1972). These infectious complications are responsible for the death of nine out of ten patients, and may be the main cause of death, even in patients with a malignancy.

Other congenital immunologic deficiencies have been associated with both susceptibility to infection and with the appearance of cancers or

16

TABLE XI.    Schematic Representation of Factors Favoring Infections
in Cancer Patients

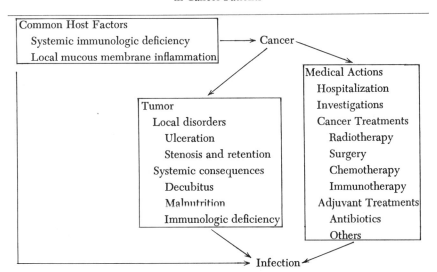

malignant blood diseases in three-quarters of the cases: these include
Wiskott-Aldrich syndrome, agammaglobulinemia, as well as various other
less-well-identified deficiencies (Kersey *et al.*, 1973).

Many other congenital diseases are accompanied by a particular susceptibility to infections and an increased risk to cancers. One has been
able to link them to an immunologic deficiency, which is not of the
utmost importance in the pathologic picture, but is nevertheless now well
identified. Among the most frequent and best studied, we shall cite
Down's syndrome (Sutnick *et al.*, 1971; Gregory *et al.*, 1972; Whittingham
*et al.*, 1977) and Chediak-Higashi disease (Wolff *et al.*, 1972).

**Acquired Abnormalities.**    Certain spontaneous immunologic deficiencies are cryptogenetic, developing in adults, and are directly linked to the
preceding situation with the same association of cancers. They are rare,
but significantly more frequent than in the normal population (Kersey
*et al.*, 1973), and frequently are superinfections (Schrub *et al.*, 1967;
Hoerni *et al.*, 1973).

Renal transplants presently constitute the most frequent cause of
acquired immune deficiency, owing to the therapeutic immunosuppression designed to prevent graft rejection. Immune deficiency thus induced
is responsible for infectious complications (Eichkhoff, 1973) and is also
linked to the development of neoplasms with a significantly increased
frequency (Hoover and Fraumeni, 1973).

Elderly patients also present poor resistance and are susceptible to increased infectious risks, owing to an immunologic deficiency which is accentuated with aging (Diaz-Jouanen *et al.*, 1975), as well as to a possibility of malignant neoplastic degeneration, which also increases with age.

Excessive alcoholic intake induces qualitative and quantitative defects which are seen *in vitro* in the thymus-derived lymphocyte population (Berenyi *et al.*, 1975; Lundy *et al.*, 1975) or *in vivo* by a cell-mediated immune response (Smith *et al.*, 1972). These defects, along with local disorders, may in part play a role in the high incidence of head and neck cancer observed in these patients.

Finally, in the same patient, fortuitous coincidences, such as diabetes (which predisposes to infections) and cancer, may be observed.

### Localized Abnormalities

Head and neck cancers usually develop in patients with poor hygienic habits. Smoking is responsible for irritation of the mucous membranes, which, even before being at the origin of cancer, maintains an inflammatory and infectious condition of variable importance that develops into characteristic chronic bronchitis. Insufficient buccodental hygiene is responsible for chronically infected stomatologic lesions. Alcoholic intoxication contributes to the maintenance of the fragility of digestive epithelium toward any aggression and also maintains general metabolic disturbances, among which immune deficiency plays a role as mentioned previously. Thus these chronically intoxicated patients have many reasons to present infections, and the addition of a neoplasm can only aggravate them. The secretion of salivary IgA is increased in smokers and in alcoholics, as well as in patients with head and neck or lung carcinoma (Mandel *et al.*, 1973), but the influence of that variation on local infections is not defined.

In all these situations, superinfections developing in a patient who has become cancerous only prolong these superinfections which had already been observed prior to the appearance of the cancer and should be primarily linked to the initial immunologic deficiency. Moreover, at the time of its appearance the cancer provides supplementary causes of infections which are particular to the cancer itself. We shall now investigate this possibility.

### TUMOR

A tumor can favor an infection either locally (by constituting a favorable culture medium for viruses, by breaking into a cutaneous or mucous lining, by a mechanical consequence) or by a systemic disturbance.

## Local Disturbances

**Intratumoral Infection.** About 10 years ago viral particles had been observed in neoplastic cells by means of electron microscopy. These observations, too often positive, rapidly led to the conclusion that the observed viruses were not responsible for cancer, but corresponded more probably to a second contamination (Dmochowski, 1960; Dmochowski *et al.*, 1976). These observations are reported here just as a reminder, for they never corresponded to a clinical infection.

**Neoplastic Ulceration.** This type of infection results from a breakdown of the natural barriers which protect the host against the external environment or the contents of septic respiratory, genital, or digestive cavities. Thus the main part of carcinomas of skin, head and neck or digestive tract, uterus, and vagina are naturally superinfected. This type of infection has hardly been studied, probably because of its banality. Thus its importance, its extension in the depth of tissues, as well as its consequences on the whole organism are unknown.

**Mechanical Consequences.** The tumor can cause the compression of various natural ducts, and thus favor an infection and obstruction to drainage above the stenosis. These phenomena can be observed for a digestive tumor or a bronchial tumor with possible formation of an abscess in the segment of the corresponding pulmonary lobe. The female urinary tract may be affected by a cervicouterine lesion, the male urinary tract by a prostatic tumor.

More indirectly, the tumor may be responsible for a pathologic fracture of a lower limb, for a paraplegia by cord compression. These conditions add to the development of decubiti and to sphincterial problems which disturb the excretory functions and constitute additional factors which favor an infection.

## General Consequences

On the whole, immunologic insufficiency that exists in the terminal stage of cancers is only due to a general deficiency of all functions of the organism (Lamb *et al.*, 1962) and probably depends on general metabolic and nutritional conditions (Gontzea, 1974). On the contrary, at earlier stages there are more specific alterations which affect humoral or cellular immunity or different phases of the inflammatory reaction, and appear in most cases as paraneoplastic manifestations (Nagel, 1971) prior to any treatment (Lehane and Lane, 1974; Lee, 1977).

**Humoral Immunity.** Globulin function is particularly disturbed during neoplasms affecting B lymphocytes whether they are secreting immunoglobulins, such as multiple myeloma or Waldenström macroglobulinemia (Mordasini *et al.*, 1972), or nonsecreting as most of the chronic lymphoid leukemias (Homberg *et al.*, 1971).

For myelomas, the production of normal immunoglobulins is reduced to 10% of the normal rate, but it can be recuperated if chemotherapy sufficiently reduces the neoplastic clone (Salmon, 1973). A balance between the two types of cellular populations, neoplastic and normal, appears to be linked to phenomena of cellular regulation, but can also depend on a metabolic competition or an interferon secretion with immunoblocking effect (Epstein and Salmon, 1974).

In other cancers immunoglobulins are normal or increased, especially in Hodgkin's disease (Wagener *et al.*, 1976). For solid tumors, the rate of immunoglobulins is usually normal, except at the terminal period of evolution (Plesničar, 1972; Roberts *et al.*, 1975). There is even an augmentation of the synthesis of antibodies, but a shortening of their half-life (Waterhouse, 1975). The humoral response to an infection is most often normal, and serodiagnosis is possible for bacterial infections (Surgalla *et al.*, 1975) or mycosis (Preisler *et al.*, 1971).

**Cell-mediated Immunity.** The impairment of cell-mediated immunity, long known for Hodgkin's disease with the negativation of the tuberculin skin test (Mantoux test), is particularly notable in this infection, but is equally present in most cancers.

Immunosuppression associated with Hodgkin's disease has been the subject of numerous studies which have been reviewed in some recent publications (Crowther, 1973; Lang, 1973; Symposium, 1973). Generally, humoral immunity is intact, except at the terminal period when the patient presents a general breakdown of all essential functions of the organism. On the contrary, cell-mediated immunity is nearly always impaired early. Agreement is far from being reached about the eventual existence of these disturbances before the appearance of the first neoplastic cells and on the recuperation of normal functions in patients with complete remission after a few years without maintenance therapy. The results of numerous analyses vary according to the technique employed and the type of patient studied. On the whole, the studies suggest, nevertheless, that the impairing of cell-mediated immunity exists as soon as the first clinical manifestation. This impairment increases either when the disease worsens, when systemic symptoms exist, or in mixed histologic forms and especially in lymphoid depletion. In a recent series of 71 patients treated for Hodgkin's disease by radiotherapy, immunologic studies show intact immunologic reactions five years after treatment and are consistent with the absence of an unusual incidence of infectious complications (Kun and Johnson, 1975). For other lymphomas, data are rarer and less clear: much more discrete deficiencies of cellular immunity have been noted in some cases and hypogammaglobulinemia in others. These modifications are quite different from those observed in Hodgkin's disease; however, they are similar to those noted during solid tumors (Miller, 1968). A recent study shows that severe immunodeficiency is found in patients with diffuse lymphoma, and definite but much less severe immunodeficiency is characteristic of patients with nodular lymphoma (Jones et al., 1977).

A deficiency of the same type, but less strong, has been recognized by the refinement of immunologic investigations for solid tumors, especially breast (Whittaker et al., 1971), lung (Han and Takita, 1972), brain (Brooks et al., 1972), gastric (Orita et al., 1976), or urogenital tumors (Schellhammer et al., 1976). Insufficiency of cell-mediated reactions can be affirmed by the study of lymphoblastic transformation by phytohemagglutinin (Sutherland et al., 1971; Barnes et al., 1975), which may be inhibited by a factor present in the serum of cancer patients (Whittaker et al., 1971; Catalona et al., 1973; Suciu-Foca et al., 1973) or by the dinitrochlorobenzene skin test (Catalona and Chretien, 1973; Bolton et al., 1975) or other skin tests (Burdick et al., 1975); whereas the tests of lymphocyte transformation have shown no difference between cancer patients and normal subjects (Levin et al., 1968). In fact, the increasingly numerous investigations to which cancer patients are submitted give variable results depending on the patient, the test employed, the type of tumor, and its stage of evolution (Golub et al., 1974; Burdick et al., 1975); thus their results are still difficult to interpret.

**Nonspecific Reactions.**    A relatively rare factor, but evident when it exists, is constituted by a leukopenia, which is generally only a part of a pancytopenia linked to bone marrow invasion. This leukopenia is observed relatively more often during leukemia, lymphoma, and dysglobulinemia, but can also be found in solid tumors at an advanced stage.

Phagocytic activity is only slightly disturbed during leukemias (Constantopoulos et al., 1973). In fact, it appears normal in patients with acute myeloid leukemia and reduced in those with acute or chronic lymphoid leukemia (Pickering et al., 1975). In another study phagocytic capabilities of granulocytes are decreased in acute myeloid leukemias and smouldering leukemias (Wilkinson et al., 1975); the lowest rate of phagocytosis is observed in untreated patients. Phagocytosis improves with chemotherapy and becomes normal in cases of complete remission; it seems that a serum factor is responsible for this impairment.

A reduction of monocytic chemotaxis has been noted for most cancer patients. It is absent in infected patients (Boetcher and Leonard, 1974) and is partially reversible with BCG administration or tumor removal (Miller, 1975).

Complement has been studied for several cancers. $C'_2$ is, on the whole, slightly increased, especially in Hodgkin's disease and multiple myeloma, but it may be decreased in some cases of non-Hodgkin's lymphomas (Southam and Siegel, 1966). Several fractions of complement have also been found to decrease during leukemias (Audran, 1970).

Interferon production may be impaired in cancer patients with advanced tumors (Rassiga-Pidot and McIntyre, 1974). On the other hand, in some cases of acute monocytic or myelomonocytic leukemia, the elevation of serum lysozyme is responsible for an increase of bacteriostatic and bactericidal activity and for a decrease in the frequency of infections (Pruzanski et al., 1973).

Leukocytic functions, evaluated by the activity of the monophosphate hexose shunt and the tetrazolium nitroblue test, are impaired in children with acute lymphoid leukemia, even during the periods of complete remission (Pickering et al., 1975).

Neutrophil migration has been the subject of numerous studies (Senn et al., 1971; Senn and Jungi, 1975). It is considerably impaired in acute leukemia, worsens under corticosteroid therapy, but is almost totally corrected in the event of a complete remission. In the myeloproliferative cancers, the moderate diminution in the early stage is aggravated with the evolution of the disease, especially during the transformation into acute leukemia. During chronic lymphoid leukemias, as well as during myelomas and malignant lymphomas, this migration is hardly disturbed, except at advanced stages of the disease.

Once the diagnosis of cancer has been formulated, the medical management introduces further disturbances which can either correct the preexisting abnormalities or aggravate them or add others.

## MEDICAL INTERVENTION

Often, and on the whole useful, medical intervention can also be the source of supplementary factors of alteration, generally temporary. This alteration can be due either to the investigations or to the treatment.

Most often, these medical interventions necessitate a hospitalization which in itself entails a risk of contamination caused by the hospital environment (hospitalism). This contamination by hospital infectious agents, a priori more pathogenic than nonhospital agents, is rarely the source of an immediate infection, but can become evident later, on the occasion of an adjunctive factor (see Chapter 3).

## Investigations

Investigations which are performed in cancer patients are rarely specific for malignant tumors. Endoscopies and catheterizations, which may be necessary, are no more hazardous for cancer than for noncancer patients.

In our experience, these investigations (endoscopies and biopsies in particular) are the source of one-quarter of the infectious complications observed in hospitalized patients in a medical service of oncology; this relative frequency is balanced by the constant benignity of these infections (Durand *et al.*, 1974).

The BCG test, designed to explore delayed hypersensitivity, is sometimes responsible for a localized inflammatory reaction in patients with severe impairment of host resistance. This complication occurred approximately once in 5000 tests in our experience. The rare severe complications caused by BCG will be discussed in Chapter 5.

Finally, lymphography, one of the most often employed investigations in cancer patients, sometimes gives a slight infection at the sites of the lymphatic injection. It may be accompanied by febrile reactions which may appear as an early reaction which is linked to the injection of the product or as a delayed reaction which is in relation to the pathologic character of the opacified lymph nodes; but these febrile reactions have never signified a superinfection (Le Treut *et al.*, 1972; Chapter 3).

## Anticancer Treatments

We shall successively look at the consequences of diverse types of treatment.

**Radiotherapy.** Radiotherapy may have a local effect by making the epithelial barrier fragile when it is accompanied by an intense epithelitis. This disorder generally remains moderate and will favor a localized and transitory infection. When cervical irradiation involves the salivary glands, it indirectly induces a xerostomia and a buccal dryness which particularly predisposes to fungal infections (Carl *et al.*, 1972). Occasionally, under the combined effect of neoplastic lesions and irradiation, a radionecrosis develops which can constitute a superinfected lesion where the infection contributes to the maintenance of the necrosis.

In the case of large abdominal irradiation, for either an ovarian, digestive, or lymphatic tumor, radiotherapy is accompanied by diffuse digestive mucositis; there is also a disturbance of the intestinal flora. Thus, general infections can be doubly enhanced.

Urinary infections are a frequent complication in the treatment of female genital cancers, often leading to obstructive lesions prior to treatment. In 167 patients treated by curietherapy, urinary infections observed in 16% of the cases before treatment became three times more frequent during and after curietherapy; this increase depended on the dose of irradiation (Widholm and Mattsson, 1972).

Systemic immunologic effects of radiotherapy have been the object of numerous observations and are the source of different viewpoints (Hoerni, 1974). Generally, irradiation determines a diminution of lymphocytosis and a reduction in the rate of lymphoblastic transformation. It seems that irradiation predominantly affects the subpopulation of T-cells which do not form high affinity E-rosettes. Irradiation of the pelvic area results in a more rapid reduction of the level of T-lymphocytes than does irradiation of the mediastinum. This reduction could be the result of radiation effects on the lymphocytes in the major blood vessels (Raben et al., 1976). In some studies a decrease in delayed hypersensitivity is found when irradiation includes the thymic area, or in Hodgkin's disease (Check et al., 1973). But for that same affection no significant modification of the BCG test following extended irradiations has been observed (Hoerni, 1974). More limited irradiations, for example, those involving head and neck fields, seem to be without effect (Gross et al., 1973). A temporary decrease of bactericidal properties of blood phagocytes has been noted following irradiation of the central nervous system in patients with acute lymphoid leukemia (Baehner et al., 1973). The largest studies have not found a regular impairment of in vivo immunologic reactions after radiotherapy (Clement and Kramer, 1974; Ghossein et al., 1975); however, a decrease of skin sensitivity can be observed in some patients, especially in those with a poor prognosis (Slater et al., 1976). On the contrary, radiotherapy can induce a hypereosinophilia, unrelated to other immunologic parameters, which is related to a good prognosis (Ghossein et al., 1975).

The relationship between radiotherapy and herpes zoster is controversial. Gremmel and Schulte-Brinkmann (1966), who have observed more than 6000 patients, find that the frequency of herpes zoster in cancer patients is the same, whether they are irradiated or not. That opinion is challenged by other authors who call attention to the fact that the localization of herpes zoster is almost always in the dermatome which corresponds to the irradiated area (Sokal and Firat, 1965; Vich, 1966); but in fact this dermatome is also the one where the tumor is and thus may have a large influence.

**Surgery.** Any operation is responsible for a rupture of the epithelial barrier. Nevertheless, aseptic conditions generally do not lead to an infectious consequence. In oncology, however, the surgeon may have to operate not only on tumors, but also in septic areas, particularly those of the digestive or respiratory tracts.

The frequency of infectious complications following cancer surgery may vary considerably depending on the site and extension of the cancer, the type of intervention performed, the surgical center and the medical team, the period considered, and also the criteria used to define infection. Systematic bacteriologic specimens demonstrate that a contamination develops during a laparotomy in one cancer patient out of two (26/50); the microorganism thus isolated is rarely responsible for a clinical infection (five cases), but postoperative infections are two times more frequent in cancer patients than in noncancer patients (Wilson *et al.*, 1974). While certain minor interventions do not seem to be followed by infectious complications, others are frequently complicated, such as, for example, Hartman's operation (Table XII). Table XII shows that the frequency of infections depends on the extent of the operation; the largest interventions are evidently linked to the maximum hazards of infection. These infections depend also on other factors such as obesity (Harris *et al.*, 1973). Meningitis and/or septicemias following craniotomy seem to be favored by the presence of an atrioventricular shunt placed prior to the operation (Naito *et al.*, 1973). Meningitis caused by *Pseudomonas* after extensive surgery for cancer of the paranasal sinuses has also been described (Geelhoed and Ketcham, 1973).

Preoperative irradiation may indirectly increase these complications: they are doubled in a series of operated breast cancers, while postoperative irradiation is without influence (Say and Donegan, 1974). In patients operated for cancer of the upper respiratory and digestive tract after irradiation, infections constitute the most frequent complication and are most often caused by *Pseudomonas*, *Staphylococcus aureus*, or *Klebsiella*. In most cases they are linked to a fistula or to a lack of healing (Smith *et al.*, 1972).

TABLE XII.   Postoperative Infections

| References | Cancer | Surgery | Infections | Comments |
|---|---|---|---|---|
| Gongaware and Slanetz (1973) | Colon and rectum | Hartmann's operation | 75% | Pelvic infections |
| Say and Donegan (1974) | Breast | Limited | 7% | Local infections |
| | | Extended | 15% | |
| Bordos *et al.* (1974) | Rectum | Limited | 17% | Local infections |
| | | Extended | 21% | |
| Harris *et al.* (1973) | Various | Inguinoiliac lymphadenectomy | 10% | Infections enhanced by obesity |

Numerous studies have been published on the infectious risks of splenectomy. Contradictory data can be essentially attributed to diverse indications for the operation and to different host situations. The fact that splenectomies have been performed recently, mainly in patients with malignant lymphomas, especially Hodgkin's disease, explains, without doubt, that numerous complications have been observed after that intervention. Some data suggest that humoral immunity is depressed by treatment in patients with Hodgkin's disease who have undergone splenectomy (Hancock et al., 1976). The splenectomy itself does not appear to run a high infectious risk, except in the young child. On the contrary, it appears that it is essentially the nature and gravity of the underlying neoplastic disease that determine the frequency and gravity of the septic complications which develop in splenectomized patients. After 92 splenectomies performed in untreated Hodgkin's disease, severe infections occurred only during marked granulocytopenia following chemotherapy (Schimpff et al., 1975). In the same series a high incidence of herpes zoster depended on the age and sex of the patients as well as on the importance of the treatment, rather than on the splenectomy itself. Treatment is also linked to the stage of the disease and thus to the importance of immunosuppression caused by cancer (Chapter 6). In the Edwards and Digioia (1976) series the incidence of infections after splenectomy also mainly depended on the severity of the underlying disease, whether this disease is neoplastic or not. However, the severity of infections is striking in splenectomized children who had Hodgkin's; moreover, Pneumococcus and Haemophilus are usually involved in these infections and Pneumoccus is responsible for septicemia or meningitis with a lethal result in half of the cases (Desser and Ultmann, 1972; Nixon and Aisenberg, 1972; Chilcote et al., 1976).

Finally, surgical interventions can lead to a slight impairment of leukocytic migration, reversible in one to three weeks (Cochran et al., 1972), as well as to other immunologic disturbances in relation either to anesthetic drugs or to the operative trauma (Howard and Simmons, 1974). The significant reduction in lymphocyte transformation seen after surgery is partly reversed in those patients transfused during the operation (Hunt and Trotter, 1976).

**Chemotherapy.**　Oncologists are utilizing drugs identical or analogous to immunosuppressive drugs, and anticancer chemotherapy can effectively have an immunosuppressive influence. However, the current method of discontinued treatment constitutes some progress, because in contrast to continuous application, it only leads to minor or no immunologic impairment. The reduction of this undesirable effect is all the more appreciable because for the same total dose the same anticancer effect is maintained

(Amiel *et al.*, 1967; Mathé *et al.*, 1969). Thus, for example, with a combination chemotherapy lasting 15 days and including a 9-day period of high dose corticosteroids, no immunologic suppression is observed in patients with Hodgkin's disease (Chauvergne *et al.*, 1973). On the contrary, a minimal dose of cyclophosphamide, methotrexate, or chlorambucil administered over a period of several weeks leads to an immune defiency (Brun, 1971) that is particularly undesirable in a cancer patient because of the infectious risk, as well as for tumoral evolution.

Nevertheless, in some particularly susceptible patients or in certain tumors having a poor response to chemotherapy, the treatment may provoke an important leukopenia which naturally favors a superinfection, as we shall again note in Chapter 3. One should remember that the number of granulocytes circulating in the blood does not accurately reflect the capability of the host which depends, above all, on the bone marrow reserve, and to a lesser degree on the marginal poor (Deinard *et al.*, 1974). This situation is especially observed in acute leukemia, where it is often necessary (particularly in the myeloid forms) to apply a treatment which induces bone marrow aplasia in order to obtain a complete remission, even a cure. The reinforcement of the treatment in acute leukemia is thus accompanied by an indisputable increase of certain infections (Perera *et al.*, 1970). It is possible that a more aggressive treatment is also justified for other tumors; it would be all the more readily applied if the risks of superinfection were better controlled.

Certain agents, such as methotrexate, and particularly 5-fluorouracil, cause lesions of the mucous membranes (especially digestive). These lesions alter the mucous membrane barrier which separates the host from a septic environment and thus create infectious portals of entry which may sometimes be very widespread (Athanassiades *et al.*, 1973).

Certain complications are caused by the method of drug introduction rather than by the drugs themselves. Thus, in a series of 210 intra-arterial infusions, 7 septicemias were observed (Marée, 1968). In another series concerning 143 infusions in 70 patients, there were 3 lethal infections (Deconti *et al.*, 1973), while another records only 0.4% superficial cutaneous infections, without systemic infection (Freckmann, 1971).

In addition, anticancer agents may have a toxic action on microorganisms, either directly or indirectly by bactericidal properties of the serum (Pruzanski and Saito, 1974). Nevertheless, it appears that the effect of this action would be, above all, to select the most resistant microorganisms (Metcalf and Hugues, 1972).

**Immunotherapy.** We shall take the opportunity to point out the risks of applying a stimulation in patients whose immunologic reactions have already been heavily taxed by the evolution of the cancer. Stimulation can then bring about an immunologic deviation, capable of exhausting the residual defenses and thus favoring infection. For this reason, among others, application of an immunologic stimulation is justified only in patients who have previously been placed in complete remission and whose tumors have been reduced as much as possible.

By all these aforementioned mechanisms the specific treatment may increase the infectious risks in cancer patients; however, it is necessary to point out the fact that when neoplastic lesions are treated, many other sources of superinfection are reduced or suppressed. We shall have the opportunity to return to this point in Chapter 9, but it is important to identify it here.

## Adjuvant Treatments

Several additional treatments may also favor a superinfection in cancer patients as they may do in any other severely or chronically ill patient.

Complications linked to the presence of intravenous or intra-arterial catheters, whether they are used for chemotherapy, parenteral alimentation, or other treatments, are well known. In a series of 93 patients fed for more than 10 days by a supraclavicular catheter, a microbial contamination of the catheter was observed in 7.3% of the cases, but only two patients showed clinical symptoms of infection (Copeland et al., 1974).

Antibiotic therapy can evidently be the source of disturbances in the resident bacterial flora and risks to select resistant microorganisms. Its utilization should thus be strictly controlled, as with any other patient. These precautions have to be emphasized and they shall be discussed later (Chapter 9).

Transfusions of blood fractions are presently less likely to carry hepatitis B virus; however, the leukocytic concentrates may be responsible for the transmission of Toxoplasma, especially when they are prepared from several donors (Siegel et al., 1971). On the other hand, blood transfusions may transmit cytomegalovirus, which is suspected of being pathogenic in immunosuppressed patients (Bussel et al., 1975).

Many medications and chemical substances, such as alcohol, can disturb phagocytic functions (Golde and Cline, 1974) and in vitro lymphocyte activity (Lundy et al., 1975). Phagocytosis may be disturbed by a hypophosphatemia owing to parental hyperalimentation (Craddock et al., 1974). Lymphoblastic transformation is reduced after simple aspirin absorption (Crout et al., 1975).

The mode of action of these diverse factors is sometimes poorly known and well defined, as we shall see in Chapter 3.

# Pathophysiology

To have an infection, the following events are required: first a microorganism, capable of becoming pathogenic, must have human contact. This microorganism can be harbored for a more or less long period or can immediately provoke an infection. For this, the microorganism must penetrate either spontaneously, or following a contaminated manipulation or a break in the epithelial covering. In some cases the debilitated patient loses normal control of microbial proliferation. These latter facts are particularly important in cancer patients.

After having considered the different stages of infection in cancer patients, we shall discuss the pathophysiology of fever, which is not always of an infectious origin in cancer patients.

## MICROBIAL CONTAMINATION

The microorganism which will provoke the infection may be spontaneously carried by the patient or may be transmitted to him.

The increased virulence of a commensal microorganism at the occasion of an intercurrent disease, especially a cancer, is a well-known notion. Numerous are the sites of the host which harbor a diversified flora, sometimes comprised of potentially very pathogenic microorganisms. These may proliferate if the patient's resistance is weakened by either traumatism or illness. It is possible, for example, to observe the influence of the normal vaginal flora on the development of infectious complications consequent to gynecologic interventions (Neary et al., 1973). The same is true for a commensal intestinal flora, whether it is Enterobacteriaceae or Candida; they may cause severe infections in immunosuppressed patients. Sometimes the starting point of the infection is not in the saprophytic flora, but rather in small or slowly evolving infectious foci (sinuses, dental, tonsillar, or gynecologic) which tend to disseminate in the same aforementioned conditions..

However, in cancer patients, these autochthonous microorganisms seem to have an ancillary role in comparison with acquired microorganisms, principally during hospitalization which is necessitated by the cancer. The bacterial flora of the oropharynx evolves and becomes enriched with Gram-negative bacilli during hospitalization. This brings about a modifi-

cation of the bacteriologic aspect of hospital contracted pneumonias. It
has thus been shown that, in an old-age home, aspiratory pulmonary infections were mainly caused by anaerobic microorganisms of the endogenous flora of Veillon, accessorily to *Streptococci* or *Pneumoccoci*; whereas
in a hospital environment the most frequent infections were no longer
caused by anaerobic microorganisms, but by *Pseudomonas* and *Enterobacteriaceae* (Lorber and Swenson, 1974). These risks of hospital contamination are well known and quite evident. Certain hospital services
are more affected than others, particularly those with severely ill patients
who constitute a favorable culture medium for diversified microbial
flora. Some services are spared, at least for a certain period, while others
are not; for example, an intensive care unit where, in addition to the
very impaired status of the patients, there are numerous manipulations
which may be sources of infection: tracheotomy, intravenous or urinary
catheters, etc. Thus, in a service of surgical reanimation almost all the
patients are colonized after 10 days and infected after 30 days of hospitalization; the length of exposure time plays an important role (Northey
*et al.*, 1974). Another study relating to 213 patients hospitalized in an
intensive care unit showed that from the first day 22% of the patients had
Gram-negative bacilli in their pharynx or sputum and that the colonization of these bacilli reached 45% by the fifth day, but never exceeded that
percentage. Out of 26 nosocomial respiratory infections, 24 were related
colonized patients and only 2 noncolonized ones (Johanson *et al.*, 1972).
On the contrary, almost all patients with acute leukemia carry Gram-
negative bacilli (in axillas and groins) on the day of their hospitalization,
while hospital staff or other cancer patients with malignant melanoma
remain free of these (McBride *et al.*, 1976).

   *Pseudomonas* has been especially studied because of the severe risks
to which it exposes cancer patients. At the moment of entry in the hospital, very few patients are colonized by this bacteria; however, half of
them will be colonized during their hospitalization (Schimpff *et al.*, 1973).
*Pseudomonas* is transmitted by the hands of the staff, alimentation, water
and ice, and various appliances of respiration, vaporization, aspiration,
etc.; sinks are unquestionable reservoirs. In addition to the medical staff
(their hands, nostrils, and clothing), the medical material (sphygmoma-
nometer, stethoscope) can also transport the bacteria. Despite the usual
precautions one cannot always avoid the entry of microorganisms by an
endoscope or a probe in an area which should remain sterile, but the risk
is especially high for in-dwelling material, such as intravenous or urinary
catheters, cannula of tracheotomy.

   Finally, without returning to the risks of operative contamination, we
shall recall the risks of transmission linked to transfusion, particularly for

leukocytic concentrates: transmission of hepatitis, toxoplasmosis, or cyto-megalovirosis.

Colonization is not necessarily followed by infection. Other factors are required.

## FROM CONTAMINATION TO INFECTION

Most infections which set in during cancers develop from the resident flora of the patient, whether or not these flora have been modified. Their modification depends on factors which are generally not well defined, except for *Pseudomonas aeruginosa* (Schimpff *et al.*, 1973). This has been particularly demonstrated for acute leukemia (Dao, 1971). In acute non-lymphoid leukemia a very regular surveyance of throat, mouth, nose, armpits, stool, and urine permits the detection of 95% of the germs re-sponsible for later infections. These infections are generally localized. They may be accompanied by a bacteremia and their development is limited to a very few places; thus, for a total of 88 infections which devel-oped in 48 patients, 20 were pulmonary, 14 anorectal, 11 cutaneous, 10 urinary, and 9 pharyngeal (Schimpff *et al.*, 1972). Thus it is necessary to envisage why one microorganism in particular, among the many which colonize a cancer patient, causes an infection.

The first reason depends on the microorganism. *Pseudomonas* is one of the bacteria which is most often involved in septicemia; this may be explained by its particular pathogenic and invading power (Schimpff *et al.*, 1973). The microorganism responsible for an infection, in cancer as well as in other patients, is determined by an antibiotic therapy, which, no matter how it is administered, selects the resistant and generally most virulent microorganism. This type of superinfection is not avoided even when broad-spectrum antibiotics are employed (Klastersky *et al.*, 1972) and in this latter case infection is often caused by fungi (see Chapter 7).

Other reasons depend on the patient and his ability to limit microbial invasion. This ability may be weakened because of an impairment of the epithelial barrier or a decrease in immunologic reactions.

The area where the epithelial covering is broken conditions the respon-sible microorganism. The same microorganism does not colonize the res-piratory tract, the digestive tract, the urinary tract, or the genital area. Thus a digestive lesion, be it neoplastic, hemorrhagic, or due to medica-tion, will, above all, favor the entry of *Pseudomonas* or *Candida* (Hughes, 1971). A digestive portal of entry is frequent for anaerobic microorgan-isms. Fungi generally enter by the respiratory tract. *Pseudomonas* is most often introduced cutaneously or by the urinary or pulmonary tract (Fish-man and Armstrong, 1972; Tapper and Armstrong, 1974). Further details

for various bacteria will be given later (see Chapter 5). We may, however, immediately emphasize that most portals of entry favor local or
locoregional infections in patients with solid tumors, while they are at
the origin of systemic or disseminated infections in patients with hematologic malignancies. In the latter patients the origin is most often intestinal and should incite an active intestinal disinfection as well as alimentary
precautions (see Chapter 9; Loiseau-Marolleau, 1970).

The general resistance of the patient is effectively no less important. We have already mentioned the frequency with which hospitalized
patients are colonized by *Pseudomonas*; but a septicemia caused by
*Pseudomonas* develops only when a severe neutropenia appears (Schimpff
*et al.*, 1973). If the infections caused by *Pseudomonas* are easy models to
observe because of their frequency, such a relationship is also possible
with other microorganisms. This leads to a discussion of the patient–
cancer–microorganism relationship.

## PATIENT–CANCER–INFECTION RELATIONSHIP

In Chapter 2 we already discussed the multiplicity of causes which
can favor the development of an infection in cancer patients. Besides the
modifications of host resistance, prior to the cancer or more often paraneoplastic, and those of microbial ecology, one may add the therapeutic
consequences on the patient as well as on the cancer and on infectious
agents. In this complex maze of pathologic relationships, it appears difficult to determine the preponderant element. To simplify the discussion
without neglecting the essential elements, one may take into account only
the main influences of the tumor and the therapy.

The fact that cancer patients are disabled in the presence of infectious agents is evident by daily experience and numerous publications
reporting such infections. There are also comparative series, limited but
convincing, which consider at the same time cancer patients and control
groups with benign diseases (Naito *et al.*, 1973; Wilson *et al.*, 1974).
There are also series with diverse types of cancers, some predisposing
more than others to infections. For example, patients with chronic myeloid leukemia (whose granulocytes may be used to treat infections in
granulocytopenic patients) have fewer infections than those who have
chronic lymphoid leukemia characterized by a hypogammaglobulinemia.

Interpretation of the observations is complicated because the risks of
infections may vary considerably for a given type of cancer, depending
on its evolutive stage, which, in turn, conditions the status of the patient
(see Chapter 11). Thus, if it is true that patients often die because they
have an infection, it is also true that they have a severe infection because
they are dying.

The influence of anticancer treatments is also difficult to discuss because these treatments are often carefully determined according to the considered cancer. In chronic lymphoid leukemia the observation that treated patients have more infections than others should not lead to the deduction that the treatment is responsible, since it is naturally applied in most cases only to patients whose leukemia is evolutive and thus determines a marked immune deficiency. The same is true when one observes that infections are more frequent in malignant lymphoma patients, treated by radiotherapy and chemotherapy, than in patients treated only by irradiation, because chemotherapy is generally applied in the most severe cases. When one observes that a scar of an extended mastectomy gets infected more often than a simple mastectomy (Say and Donegan, 1974), one must remember that the size of the incision depends generally on the tumoral extension. For some authors, infections observed in cancer patients are linked to cancer chemotherapy, just as infections observed in patients having transplants are linked to immunosuppressive therapy. But this analogy is inaccurate, for, despite the analogies of drugs, anticancer chemotherapy, far from aiming at immunosuppression, seeks to avoid it and sometimes succeeds perfectly. However, one cannot overlook the toxic effects of a treatment. In a homogeneous series of acute leukemias, it has been possible to demonstrate that a supplementary therapy does not improve the anticancer efficacy, but adds to the toxicity by substantially increasing infectious complications (Berry et al., 1975). Moreover, the action of these treatments on host resistance remains difficult to define, owing to the difficulty of interpreting the immunologic investigations, which do not always give concurring results, owing to the associations with the immune modifications linked to cancer. In children with diverse cancers in remission, the infections were significantly correlated to a neutropenia, a hypogammaglobulinemia, and an impairment of the cell-mediated immune response (absent or very limited in noninfected children), but the origin of these immunologic disturbances has not been precisely defined (Graham-Pole et al., 1975).

After these remarks which lead to a pathophysiologic interpretation, it seems possible to sort out four types of patient–cancer–infection relationships, depending on the types of cancer and conditioning the types of infection (Table XIII).

The most frequent situation corresponds to solid tumors, which are the large majority, for they represent more than 90% of all cancers. We have seen in Chapter 2 that in these patients detailed immunologic investigations allow the detection of an impairment of delayed hypersensitivity which is inconstant and moderate, while humoral immunity remains intact, except at an advanced stage of the tumor. At the origin of an infec-

TABLE XIII. Physiopathology of Main Infections in Cancer Patients

| Cancers | Disorders | Infections |
|---|---|---|
| Solid Tumors | Local disorders: ulceration, stenosis, retention<br>Mild systemic immune deficiency | Local infections due to local lesions with occasional systemic dissemination |
| Multiple myeloma and chronic lymphocytic leukemia<br>Malignant lymphomas | Immunoglobulin deficiency | Bacterial infections, especially of respiratory tract |
| Hodgkin's disease: Early | Cellular immunologic deficiency plus immunoglobulin deficiency | Viral infections plus bacterial infections and mycosis |
| Late | Few immunologic disorders | Few infections |
| Non-Hodgkin's lymphoma | Immunologic disorders | Severe infections: septicemias, generalized viral and fungal infections |
| Acute leukemias | Granulocytopenia | |

tion the main role seems to be played by local consequences of the cancer, particularly mechanical. The infections almost always have a direct anatomic relation with the tumor. Generally, it is an infection of either a neoplastic ulceration or of the area above a neoplastic stenosis. Thus one observes, in particular, urinary infections in compressive cancers of the pelvis or respiratory infections in cancers of the bronchi or upper respiratory tract. When a treatment by radiation or surgery is applied, it also can favor locoregional infections. Patients with solid tumors are rarely submitted to an aggressive chemotherapy which causes bone marrow aplasia. The chemotherapy, nevertheless efficacious, that they usually receive does not particularly cause infections. For these tumors as well as for the treatment, the main risks probably come from antibiotic treatment. This is the reason why most mycotic infections are observed in cancer patients who had been previously submitted to antibiotics (see Chapter 7). In two series of bacteremia caused by *Pseudomonas*, more patients were under antibiotics than under anticancer chemotherapy (Fishman and Armstrong, 1972; Iannini *et al.*, 1974). The more particularly unfavorable role of broad-spectrum antibiotics has been recognized (Klastersky *et al.*, 1972). The inutility of antibiotics given prophylactically is now established (see Chapter 9) and in addition, they risk the favoring of a selection of resistant microorganisms and thus cause the appearance of severe infections. The application of antibiotics should thus be carefully limited and controlled.

Malignant blood diseases present quite a different situation because they have marked immunologic paraneoplastic consequences. The influence of this immunosuppression on the development of infections is clear: they are often generalized and with a few exceptions the blood malignancy is of no value on the infectious localization. Some of them justify aggressive chemotherapy and lead to severe leukopenia which directly determines particularly severe and disseminated infections. These quite different mechanisms are realized by systemic lymphoproliferative diseases, Hodgkin's lymphomas, and acute leukemias.

Systemic lymphoproliferative diseases are mainly represented by multiple myeloma and chronic lymphoid leukemia. In multiple myeloma the insufficiency of normal immunoglobulins is the most marked and its kinetics have been most carefully studied: it is aggravated by the cancer and is capable of recuperating when the tumoral population is reduced by anticancer therapy (Sullivan and Salmon, 1972). This hypogammaglobulinemia is less marked but constant for chronic lymphoid leukemia while the delayed hypersensitivity is always normal at the time of diagnosis Bernadou *et al.*, 1971). The relative disturbances of the lymphoblastic transformation tests (Block *et al.*, 1969) actually express only the dilution of normal lymphoid cells in the neoplastic population (most often involving B lymphocytes). Thus patients with these diseases mainly suffer bacterial infections, naturally more frequent during myeloma than during lymphoid leukemia (Twomey, 1973). For these cancers the particular importance of respiratory infections comes from the preponderant role of the secretory immunoglobulins in the protection of the corresponding mucous membrane. The elective preventive treatment of these infections is an efficacious anticancer treatment (see Chapter 8), which is the best way to correct the paraneoplastic insufficiency of the immunoglobulins.

Malignant lymphomas afford a striking contrast between Hodgkin's disease (where the paraneoplastic immune deficiency is important) and non-Hodgkin's lymphomas (where it is discrete, and close to that observed in solid tumors). This is the reason why infectious complications are observed predominantly in Hodgkin's disease (Durand et al., 1972). Contrary to what is observed in chronic lymphoid leukemia, immunologic impairment is here elective of delayed hypersensitivity and related to viral infections, particularly herpes zoster. One may also note that some infections, which are particularly observed in Hodgkin's patients, are caused by Listeria monocytogenes, against which a cellular reaction mainly intervenes. In addition, these infections are more often seen when the immune deficiency is marked, especially in the histologic forms of lymphoid depletion (Hoerni et al., 1971; Durand et al., 1972; Monfardini et al., 1973). The cell-mediated immunologic impairment may become complicated at an advanced stage of the illness by a humoral insufficiency, which one may consider as being related to the generalization of herpes zoster since the diminution of serum antibodies seems to favor the dissemination of the virus in the blood stream (Fauconnier, 1972). The unfavorable prognostic influence of the viral infection is only due to the alteration of the patient's status in relation to his cancer (see Chapter 11).

Acute leukemias offer a mixed picture. An alteration in the phagocytic function of the granulocytes exists spontaneously in myeloid forms and appears in relapsing lymphoid forms (Pickering et al., 1975). Prior to treatment, cellular immunity is hardly disturbed and humoral immunity is normal. The induction treatment reduces the synthesis of antibodies, but respects delayed hypersensitivity, except if it brings about bone marrow aplasia (Dupuy et al., 1971). During maintenance treatment, immunity is hardly impaired but it may be altered by reinduction chemotherapy. When this treatment is discontinued, one observes a recovery of normal immunoglobulins in patients remaining in complete remission, while, in cases of relapses, the immunoglobulins are not modified (Ragab et al., 1970). These data show well the interplay between the effects of treatment and the consequences of the illness. All the factors become very unfavorable for acute nonlymphoid leukemia in which complete remission is often obtained only at the price of bone marrow aplasia. It is at this time that the neutropenia, almost always less than 500 and generally 100 granulocytes/mm³, constitutes the main element triggering a severe infection, usually a septicemia, developing from a microorganism that the patient was harboring without inconvenience until that time (Frei *et al.*, 1965; Bodey *et al.*, 1966; Schimpff *et al.*, 1973; Atkinson *et al.*, 1974). Thus the prognosis of these infections depends mainly on the bone marrow status which in turn conditions a granulocytic recovery, more or less rapid and complete (Atkinson *et al.*, 1974).

This schematic presentation of cancer–infection relations, simplified and limited to specific and indisputable aspects, should not ignore (1) the possibility, in any cancer patient, of an intercurrent infection owing to chance; (2) the risks of contamination linked to hospitalization; (3) the hazards of the treatment; and (4) finally, all infections, particularly fungal, which appear at the terminal period of evolution of cancers, as in all debilitating and fatal illnesses. During the terminal evolution, which is observed in most uncurable cancers, there are, in addition, the consequences of denutrition, of global immunosuppression, of long bed-ridden periods, and even of treatment.

At this stage, as in others, one finds the initial responsibility of the cancer which directly or indirectly conditions the weakening of the patient's host defense mechanisms, the necessary treatments, and the alteration of the antimicrobial defenses. This explains why the gravity of the cancer is often recognized as the main prognostic factor for the evolution of a secondary infection (Klastersky *et al.*, 1972).

## FEVER IN CANCER PATIENTS

Fever, a symptom common both to cancers and to infections, raises diagnostic problems which shall be discussed in Chapter 4. Here we shall discuss only the principal mechanisms which may cause fever in cancer patients and which are similar to general mechanisms of fever. Fever is the consequence of a disorder in the thermoregulation center, either by a direct action of a mechanical or a metabolic factor or by an indirect action which involves pyrogen substances. These pyrogens may themselves be the result of an inflammatory reaction or a delayed hypersensitivity phenomenon with a leukocytic origin. They also may come from bacteria or be produced by a cellular necrosis, eventually tumoral (Table XIV).

### *Paraneoplastic Fevers*

Known for a long time, their direct relationship with neoplastic proliferation, although probably complex and poorly understood, is now well described (Silver, 1963). Their regression with an efficacious and usually

TABLE XIV.   Physiopathology of Fever in Cancer Patients

| | |
|---|---|
| I. Fever due to Cancer (Paraneoplastic Fever) | |
| Pyrogens | Kidney, liver cancers |
| Inflammation | Evolutive cancers |
| Immunologic reactions | Hodgkin's disease |
| Metabolic disorders | Miscellaneous |
| Direct action on | Brain tumors |
| thermoregulation centers | |
| II. Fever due to Infections | |
| Pyrogens synthesized by infectious agents or by granulocytes | |
| III. Other Fevers | |
| Thrombosis | BCG therapy |
| Metabolic disorders | Antibiotics |
| Anemia | Blood products |
| Lymphography | Miscellaneous |
| Chemotherapy | |

complete treatment of the cancer, and only with it, constitutes the proof. Malignant blood diseases and especially Hodgkin's disease are often responsible for fever, but many solid tumors, particularly those of the kidney and liver, may also be responsible. The case of fever linked to renal cancer which completely disappears on the evening of the nephrectomy and reappears at the same time as a metastasis, which again disappears after a complete removal of one isolated metastase, is too classical to be disputed (Bodel, 1974).

Even when the relationship between fever and cancer is indisputable, its mechanism still remains questionable.

Since the existence of pyrogen substances has been shown in fever in general (Wolstenholme and Birch, 1971), as well as the synthesis of diverse secretions in tumoral cells, the most simple explanation is in that of a secretion of pyrogen substances by the tumor. This pyrogen may not be secreted, but may be released by a tumoral lysis during a spontaneous necrosis or under the influence of the treatment. Such a substance has been found in the urine of Hodgkin's patients (Sokal and Shimaoka, 1967). Its protein nature is probable, because of the suppression of fever under the influence of agents inhibiting protein synthesis (Young and Dowling, 1975).

The action of an inflammatory reaction has been suggested by the variations of a chemotaxis inactivator (Ward and Berenberg, 1974) and appears particularly probable in the case of neoplastic effusions, in which the anaerobic environment favors the release of pyrogens by the leukocytes (Moore *et al.*, 1970). Such aseptic inflammatory reactions could cause the intervention of pyrogens secreted not by neutrophil granulocytes, but by monocytes (Bodel and Atkins, 1967). In Hodgkin's disease, the passage of antigenic neoplastic cells in the blood stream is probably the source of a generalized immunologic febrile reaction of a delayed hypersensitivity type which agrees with other immunologic data and the evolution of the disease (Hoerni *et al.*, 1970).

An inflammatory reaction appears particularly evident for certain cancers with a rapid evolution: fever around 38°C (100°F) without a precise cause is very often accompanied by rapid tumoral growth and poor prognosis. This inflammatory reaction is easily demonstrated in certain breast cancers by the clinical or thermographic data in the immediate neighborhood of the tumor; and since their metastatic potential is known, one can allow a diffuse reaction of this type at the origin of fever, but this does not aid in its comprehension.

A general metabolic process which alters cerebral cells appears to be involved when fever is accompanied by a paraneoplastic syndrome of hypercalcemia or by a syndrome of inappropriate ADH secretion (Schwartz–Bartter syndrome).

Lastly, some primary brain tumors or intracranial metastasis may have a direct action on the thermoregulation centers.

## Infectious Fevers

These are probably more frequent than paraneoplastic fevers. They may be related to leukocytic pyrogens. In most cases endogenous pyrogens are elaborated by the neutrophil granulocytes under the influence of bacterial products. However, fever may be observed, even in the absence of leukocytes, in infected patients with bone marrow aplasia. Knowledge about pyrogens, particularly about the lipopolysaccharides which are directly dependent on microorganisms, enables this observation to be comprehended.

## Other Fevers

Cancer patients are exposed, in addition to infections, to other complications which may cause fever; for example, venous thrombosis or a state of dehydration that certainly requires particular attention.

Anemia sometimes appears responsible for a moderate hyperthermia which may be corrected by transfusions. A pancytopenia may also be complicated by fever, even if it is not possible to relate it to an infectious complication.

Consequent to lymphangiography, a febrile period is often observed.

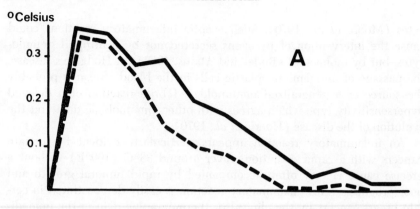

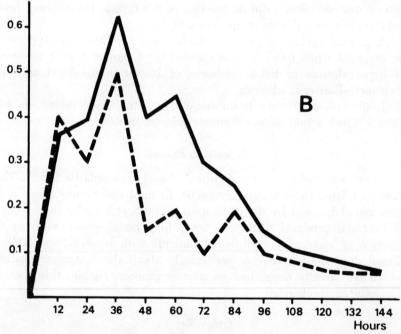

**Fig. 1.** Mean febrile reaction after lymphography in 192 patients with malignant lymphoma. The thermic ascent is significantly ($p < 0.001$) more marked after large dose injection of oiled contrast medium (B) than after small doses (A). The delayed reaction (after 36 hr) is also significantly ($p < 0.001$) more marked in patients with an abnormal lymphography (—) than in patients with a normal lymphography (---) (from Le Treut et al., 1972).

This fever is moderate and temporary, without any infection of the small incision at the site of the lymphatic catheterization. Most often, it seems

linked to the administration of the oily contrast medium which is particularly responsible for a relatively small, but diffuse pulmonary emboli
whose importance is related to that of the fever (Bjorn-Hansen and
Hagen, 1970; Le Treut et al., 1971). Moreover, in the case of malignant
lymphomas, this febrile reaction has been broken down into two elements: (1) an early reaction which mainly depends on the injected contrast medium and its quantity; (2) a late reaction that is correlated to
the tumoral abnormalities of the opacified lymph nodes, which might
depend on the release of neoplastic pyrogen by-products in the circula-
tory system (Fig. 1).

Anticancer treatments may, in some cases, be accompanied by fever.
Fever observed during, or as a consequence of, irradiation may be related
to a tumoral lysis and to a release of various metabolites into the organism or sometimes to an important inflammatory reaction, especially in the
mediastinum. Certain chemotherapeutic drugs, like cytarabine or bleomycin, may bring about rapid febrile reactions. For bleomycin, they
appear significantly more marked in Hodgkin's patients than in other
cancer patients (E.O.R.T.C., 1972). For other drugs, like asparaginase,
fever is due to a hypersensitivity reaction when the drug is given for the
second time. Immunostimulation by BCG applied in large scarifications
may also, in the next 24 hr, provoke a generalized reaction owing to the
passage of the bacilli into the blood stream and hence to a systemic inflammatory reaction. These febrile reactions are much more marked after
intratumoral injection of BCG (Sparks et al., 1973).

The responsibility of other treatments (antibiotics or various other
drugs) may sometimes be questionable in cancer patients as well as in
other subjects. Posttransfusion febrile reactions suggest that irregular
auto- or isoantibodies should be looked for so that particular precautions
can be taken to ensure that a perfect transfusion compatibility is assured
in cancer patients.

# CHAPTER 4

# General Diagnostic Problems

Sometimes infections reveal the existence of a cancer. Most often they develop during the course of a known solid tumor or hematologic neoplasm. The diagnosis of these infections raises diverse difficulties which vary with the nature of the underlying cancer and its stage, and also with the nature of the causal agent and the anatomical site of the infection.

The cancer which favors the infection also produces the clinical features which may be a source of diagnostic difficulties. Frequently, the infections are localized at the site of or in close proximity to solid tumors, while they are often generalized in the course of hematologic malignancies and severe granulocytopenias. The locations of the infections are easily identified when the solid tumor is localized or when hematologic malignancies are in remission. On the other hand, they usually become more subtle, with few clinical manifestations, and are sometimes discovered only at necropsy when the cancer is advanced or has terminated causing the death of the patient.

Bacterial infections are by far more frequent than mycosis and parasitosis. Specific microbiologic diagnosis of these infections, regardless of their nature, raises some difficulties of realization and/or interpretation; but the treatment depends on this identification and, as we shall see later, infections are a primordial element in the evolution and prognosis of cancer patients.

We shall successively consider the clinical circumstances which raise suspicion about infectious complications and the appropriate microbiologic examinations needed for diagnosis.

## CLINICAL DIAGNOSIS

During the evolution of a cancer the pathologic manifestations linked to the neoplastic process must be distinguished from those linked to intercurrent complications: infection, thromboembolism, side effects of anticancer therapy, or sometimes even of antibiotic therapy. This distinction is not always evident. For example, the computed tomography appearance of methotrexate-induced leucoencephalopathy is indistinguishable from that of a brain abscess (Bjorgen and Gold, 1977).

Regular clinical follow-up of cancer patients is essential for choosing appropriate laboratory investigations. An infection is suspected either by the observation of systemic symptoms (the main one being fever), by the presence of visceral manifestations, or because there are evident portals of entry. However, the clinical characteristics of these infections are often altered or even misleading in cancer patients, particularly when there is severe granulocytopenia. The clinical picture is even more complicated because several infections can evolve simultaneously and can be mixed with other intercurrent complications in generalized solid tumors as well as in hematologic malignancies which resist therapy.

These general notions lead to a discussion on the following points: (1) the signification of fever; (2) the importance of researching the portals of entry; (3) the problems arising from focal infections which may be either the cause or the consequence of dissemination in septicemia.

## Signification of Fever

A urinary or respiratory infection occurring concurrently with a solid tumor does not always lead to a thermic reaction, but the common denominator of nearly all infections in cancer is fever (Lacut et al., 1974). Fever is not, however, always of an infectious origin in a cancer patient and its cause is sometimes difficult to ascertain. At its genesis the hyperthermic role of certain cancers, as well as thromboembolism and applied treatments, must not be excluded; these different causes are often combined (see Chapter 3).

In a series of 526 cases composed of 2/3 solid tumors and 1/3 hematologic malignancies, a febrile status was observed in 344 patients (63.4%) (Lacut et al., 1974). One hundred and twenty times out of 344 (36.6%) fever existed prior to hospitalization, thus many patients were admitted directly in an infectious disease service. The fever lasted, on the average, 12 days for hospitalized patients, while the mean fever duration was 25 days for all patients; only 49 patients had a pyrexia of more than 20 days. One hundred and three times the fever was expressed by a short isolated attack, 108 times an intermittent course, 120 times a continuous way, and 13 times the fever curve was complex. There are 384 causes of fever in 344 patients because the same patient sometimes had two or three successive febrile episodes. An infectious origin was recorded in 146 case histories and appeared to be mainly bacterial; most often it was an isolated or an intermittent febrile manifestation. A fever specifically linked to a tumor or to a hematologic neoplasm was affirmed in 136 cases by convergent clinical and biological arguments. Twenty-six times the febrile reaction was considered to be due to particular causes, such as thromboembolism, lymphography, or transfusions. Finally, in 76 patients (20%), a precise cause was not found. It is interesting to note that the duration of fevers of "unknown origin" was less than 5 days in three-quarters of the cases and less than 10 days in 93% of the cases; it seem logical to assume that some of them were related to passing viruses.

For a total of 100 febrile episodes in 56 granulocytopenic patients (with less than 1000 granulocytes/mm³) having acute leukemia or bone marrow aplasia, Atkinson et al. (1974) were able to explain the pyrexia in 68 cases: 58 times an infection was responsible (30 were septicemias), only 2 times was a paraneoplastic process responsible. In this series there is again a high proportion of fevers of "unknown origin" (32 cases).

Any cancer may produce fever. It is more common among the digestive (colon, stomach, pancreas, and liver), female genital, pulmonary, or upper respiratory cancers than in breast, kidney, ovary, and thyroid cancers: 66% for the colon and the rectum; 44% for the liver and bile tract; 41% for the stomach; 36% for the uterus (Boggs and Frei, 1960). Superinfection causes the large majority of the febrile reactions during cancers of hollow organs, such as the digestive or respiratory tracts, but is is also particularly frequent in lymphomas and leukemias. The paraneoplastic fevers observed during lymphomas often have prolonged febrile periods which may last several months in some cases. They may very well simulate fevers derived from infectious foci (Aubertin and Aubertin, 1963; Aubertin et al., 1974).

There is still no decisive feature which differentiates an infectious from a neoplastic fever. It is the clinical context and the paraclinical examinations which guide the diagnosis. Infections and/or cancers may be obscured under the aspects of prolonged febrile periods during which the clinical examination does not show any abnormalities. The etiologic diagnosis is affirmed only by diverse investigations composed mainly of bacteriologic research and radiologic examinations (cholecystography, cholangiography, intravenous pyelography, lymphography, abdominal arteriography), and even laparotomy (Ben-Shosan et al., 1971). Thus, for 303 prolonged and duly identified febrile periods, Aubertin et al. (1974) found an isolated infection in 54% of the cases and a cancer in nearly 30% of the cases with an occasional superinfection, which might explain the thermic reaction. In a series of 36 patients with cancer who met the classical criteria for fever of an unknown origin, 18 patients also had infections, while in the other 18 only the neoplasm appeared responsible for the fever (Luft et al., 1976).

The fever may be integrated in a clinical context which immediately raises suspicion of a focal infection or a viral systemic infection; moreover, the local manifestations are sometimes the source of diagnostic difficulties.

In other circumstances it is a fortuitous observation or careful research of a portal of entry which elucidates a fever by focal infection or septicemia.

## Portal of Entry

It is rare that viral or parasitic infections are suspected by their site of entry, as they enter the organism by the upper digestive or respiratory tract, often by means of microscopic lesions. Rarely, the history of transfusions or parenteral injections may suggest a viral hepatitis or cytomegalic inclusion disease.

However, the existence of a portal of entry is useful for the diagnosis of a bacterial or fungal infection. The existence of an intravenous catheter, particularly if it is responsible for local inflammatory phenomena, suggests a bacterial or fungal septicemia, and requires blood cultures to determine an appropriate treatment. The same is true for postoperative fevers; most of them originate from an infectious complication and can be due to either a superficial or deep suppuration or a septicemia.

Moreover, an ulcerated cancer constitutes a potential portal of entry, for example, in the upper respiratory tract. It is evident that cancers of the pharynx, larynx, and bronchi predispose to bacterial pneumonias (sometimes complicated by pleural effusions), as do those of the urogenital tract to urinary infections.

All febrile conditions in cancer patients, either in the absence or even in the presence of focal manifestations, are mainly caused by bacterial infections, particularly septicemia. Blood cultures as well as systematic cultures of the natural microbial foci (mouth, pharynx, stool, urine) should be undertaken; however, these results must be interpreted as we shall discuss further on.

## Localized Infections

More than 90% of cancers are solid tumors and develop near cavitary organs. This leads to local manifestations which are exposed to bacterial superinfections; moreover, these local infections are favored by radiotherapy, curietherapy, and surgery (see Chapter 2). Infectious phenomena may also be found elsewhere than at the site of the initial cancer. Thus it is sometimes difficult to determine the metastatic or infectious nature of some complications.

Certain localized infections raise particular diagnostic difficulties which differ depending on whether the diagnosis of cancer has been established or not.

**Pleuropulmonary Manifestations.**  The discussion of the nature of a single pulmonary lesion arises especially during bronchogenic carcinoma when the infectious process mainly involves a hypoventilated and poorly vascularized area situated above the tumoral stenosis. Sometimes the diagnosis of cancer has been established and sometimes the suppurative syndrome is the first episode of the clinical history. In this case, the elements which suggest a cancer are the direct retractile character of the lobar opacity and the poor response to the anti-infectious treatment. However, some pulmonary suppurations which develop above a tumoral stenosis may react very well to antibiotics and be completely cleared. The suppuration of a necrosed cancer mass is much rarer (Fig. 2); this condition is especially found in peripheral bronchogenic cancers, rarely in secondary pulmonary cancers. All these superinfections are frequent during bronchogenic carcinomas and they relapse readily owing to the maintenance of the stenosis before the diagnosis of cancer is established and the treatment is applied.

In addition, bacterial pneumopathies, in particular those caused by *Pneumococcus*, may take a rather long time to have their radiologic abnormalities disappear, even without an underlying cancer. These pneumonic radiographic abnormalities regress in 6 weeks in patients less than 50 years old, nonalcoholic, and without an obstructive bronchopathy; in 14 weeks in patients who are older and exempt from defects. Alcoholism and chronic degenerative bronchial alterations evidently increase the delay of resolution of the infectious lesions (Jay *et al.*, 1975).

Multiple nonsystematized pulmonary images may be related to a bacterial or tuberculous bronchopneumonia and also to a virus or infection such as candidiasis, aspergillosis, or pneumocystosis. However, they are sometimes the consequence of leukemic infiltrates, lymphoma localizations, or pulmonary metastasis.

Although uncommon, pulmonary alveolar proteinosis may be associated with blood malignancy (18 cases of such an association have been reported; Delarue *et al.*, 1969; Carnovale *et al.*, 1977). Different radiologic abnormalities caused by proteinosis are usually difficult to distinguish either from specific tumoral localization or from infections, all the more so as infection is often superimposed to proteinosis.

The analysis of the clinical and radiographic data is important, but generally not sufficient. The precise answer often comes only from the laboratory data, but sometimes only after special examinations, such as a pulmonary biopsy.

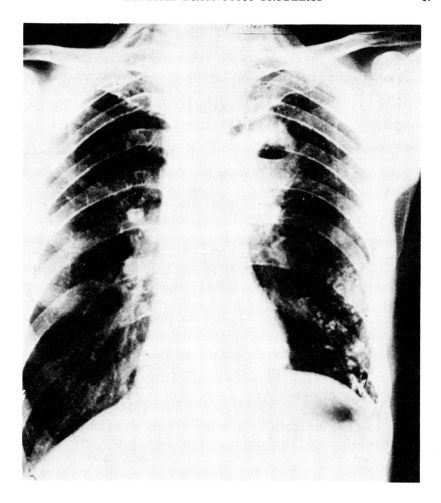

**Fig. 2.** Lung epidermoid carcinoma with central necrosis and superinfection.

A pleural effusion often evokes a neoplastic pleuritis related to a cancerous lesion of the serous membrane or to the inflammation provoked by a neighboring parenchymous tumoral extension, especially if it has a hemorrhagic and recurring character. However, when the pleural fluid has a serofibrinous aspect and does not contain abnormal cells, the diagnosis may be subject to further speculation. Thus, for the latter pleuritis, when it is paucisymptomatic, subacute, or of chronic evolution, tuberculosis should be considered; when it is acute, with functional signs, a viral infection or even a pulmonary embolism should be kept in mind for the diagnosis.

**Digestive and Hepatic Manifestations.** Diarrhea and acute dysenteric syndromes in cancer patients rarely cause diagnostic difficulties; they are generally of infectious origin, either bacterial, viral, or parasitic. Sometimes they are the side effects of antibiotics, of anticancer chemotherapy (5 fluorouracil), of abdomino-pelvic radiotherapy, or of gynecologic or vesical curiethreapy. On the other hand, a prolonged diarrhea should not be too easily related to an infection; one should be vigilant in looking for colon cancer which sometimes manifests itself in that way at the beginning.

Jaundice is a common manifestation during cancer. Most often it is due to hepatitis or cholestasis. Cancer patients, submitted to injections, blood tests, or transfusions, may be victims of serum hepatitis, but anticancer chemotherapy may sometimes be toxic for hepatic cells and may induce cytolytic hepatitis (Berthelot *et al.*, 1965). Straightforward, progressive, and painless cholestatic jaundice evokes a compression or an invasion of the biliary tract by a cancer, but when it is moderate or stable, one may envisage a cholestatic viral hepatitis or a hepatitis related to the prolonged utilization of estrogens or progestins (used in the treatment of hormone-dependent tumors). Finally, a specific infiltration of the liver parenchyma by Hodgkin's disease can bring about mixed syndromes of cytolysis and moderate cholestasis which may clinically be revealed by jaundice of a variable intensity.

**Lymph-node Manifestations.** A lymphadenopathy which is superficial, cold, hard, well limited, and painless is sometimes not tumoral but tuberculous. The incomplete regression of cervical lymphadenopathies consequent to repeated mild sore throats should be considered as suspect and sometimes leads to the discovery of a neoplastic pathology, such as throat cancer or Hodgkin's disease (Hoerni *et al.*, 1971). Micropolyadenopathies, symptomatic of toxoplasmosis, are sometimes biopsied because of the suspicion of Hodgkin's disease if the serodiagnosis of toxoplasmosis has been omitted; but the association of these two diseases can be encountered.

**Cutaneous Manifestations.** The extremely polymorphous cutaneous manifestations of infections are most often related to their cause. Sometimes subcutaneous nodules, more or less inflammatory with an aspect of erythema nodosum, are considered to be due to an infection or an immunologic reaction, while they are actually due to a neoplastic process. Uncharacterized nonspecific skin lesions such as hemorrhagic phenomena, pruritus, urticaria, papules, vesicles, subcutaneous nodules, and erythema multiforme are sometimes described in patients with acute myelogenous leukemia (Klock and Oken, 1976).

**Meningeal Manifestations.** A subacute meningitis with intracranial hypertension, eventual neurologic focused symptoms, and a mixed or lymphocytic celular reaction of the cerebrospinal fluid may be due either to *Mycobacterium, Listeria,* a fungus, or also to meningeal carcinosis.

**Other Localizations.** Dysphagia in a cancer patient presents a diagnostic challenge: candidiasis is the most common cause of esophagitis, but there are other causes of dysphagia such as viruses, chemotherapy, radiation, esophageal tumor, motility disorders, or gastric reflux (Lightdale *et al.,* 1977.

Other manifestations, such as urinary infections, generally do not cause major difficulties, except for deep suppurations. Figure 3 illustrates some diagnostic problems raised by skeletal lesions.

### Particular Cases of Malignant Blood Diseases and Severe Granulocytopenias

Bacterial, as well as viral, mycotic, and parasitic infections, are characterized by their severity, their diffusion, and their tendency to generalize. Moreover, some of them, such as cryptococcosis and pneumocystosis, practically appear only during malignant blood diseases and in immunosuppressed patients.

The frequency and gravity of infections during severe granulocytopenias have been demonstrated. The bacterial risk appears when the number of granulocytes falls lower than 1500/mm$^3$, but is especially important below 1000 and practically constant below 500. Moreover, it is all the more marked when the granulocytopenia lasts a long time. In patients with acute leukemia, 90% of the disseminated mycoses and 78% of the septicemias develop when the level of granulocytes is lower than 500/mm$^3$; moreover, 60% of the patients with less than 1000 neutrophil granulocytes become infected in 3 weeks time (Bodey *et al.,* 1966). The myelotoxic drugs certainly contribute to increasing the risk and duration of granulocytopenia.

The absence of neutrophil granulocytes, thus of phagocytosis, brings about particular aspects of the infectious foci: the inflammatory reaction is disturbed and the microorganisms multiply without producing pus. This is the reason why local and generalized manifestations have been very much studied and quantified (for pharyngeal, anorectal, cutaneous, urinary, and pulmonary infections) according to the number of granulocytes/mm$^3$ (less than 100; between 100 and 1000; more than 1000). It has been demonstrated that exudations, collections with or without fluctuation, ulcerations or fistulizations, and reactions of the regional

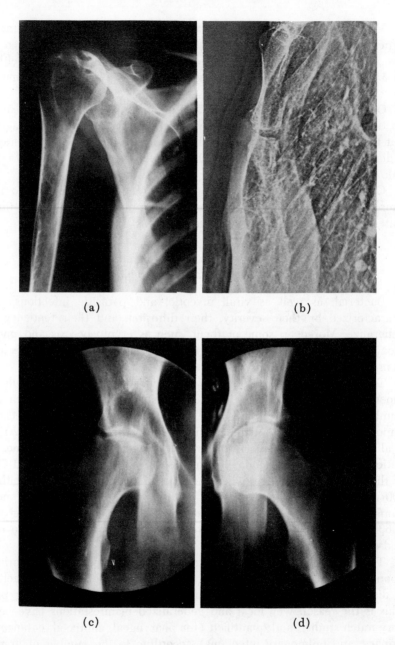

(a)         (b)

(c)         (d)

**Fig. 3.** A 43-year-old woman exhibiting advanced Hodgkin's disease with four types of osseous lesions: (*a*) humeral osteolytic lesions of undetermined origin; (*b*) Hodgkin's sternal lesion; (*c*) right hip joint lesion considered as due to aseptic osteonecrosis but actually due to Salmonella osteoarthritis; (*d*) left hip joint aseptic osteonecrosis probably favored by corticosteroids.

lymph nodes were less frequent when granulocytopenia was more pronounced, while bacteremias and fever were more common in the same conditions (Sickles et al., 1975). In these conditions extended lesions of pulmonary parenchyma can occur without expectoration and urinary infections with little dysuria and without leukocyturia. The virulence of the microorganisms sometimes causes infarctions and ischemic necrosis (secondary to arterial invasion). These clinical consequences shall be discussed later.

Pulmonary manifestations are the most frequent visceral lesions. Acute interstitial pneumonias in the immunosuppressed host are frequent and often lethal (Armstrong, 1976). A tachypnea, as well as a cyanosis, is sometimes the warning sign in a febrile patient. The physical pulmonary examination may be asymptomatic and the radiography (which should systematically be done in these cases) shows a more or less diffuse pneumopathy. A positive correlation was found between the granulocyte count and the presence of radiographic abnormalities; the different types of organisms could not be distinguished by the radiographic appearance (Zorzona et al., 1976) and sometimes the parenchymous lesion is shown only by necropsy. "Necrotizing pneumopathy," which is particular to agranulocytosis, shows in a few days a sequestrum encircled by a limiting sulcus (Camilleri and Diebold, 1972). These infections are very grave, being lethal in 80% of the cases (Dao, 1975). The responsible microorganisms are predominantly bacteria, but Candida, Aspergillus, Pneumocystis, and even Cytomegalovirus are also found. The etiologic diagnosis of these infections is difficult and not always established during the lifetime of the patient; it is also sometimes difficult to distinguish from neoplastic pulmonary infiltrations or from pulmonary fibrosis caused by busulfan, bleomycin, cyclophosphamide, or methotrexate. Bronchowashings and bronchial brushing have thus been proposed to find the responsible microorganism; transtracheal biopsies cannot be done when hemostatic troubles exist (owing essentially to thrombocytopenia).

Other infectious localizations are well described. Necrotizing pharyngitis, ulceronecrotic stomatitis, even dental infections, are well known. Among the gastrointestinal lesions, certain of them which are minimal and imperceptible are responsible for septicemias, others are symptomatic such as perianal or perirectal abscesses; finally, one should mention necrotizing enterocolitis which has a complex pathogenesis in which bacterial or fungal infection intervenes and evolves toward perforation and death (Steinberg et al., 1973).

Urinary tract infections cause few or no symptoms and may or may not lead to pyuria. Cutaneous bacterial lesions are sometimes necrotic, such as ecthyma gangrenosum due in some cases not only to Pseu-

*domonas* but also to *Enterobacteriaceae* (Dao, 1975) or *Aeromonas* (Ketover *et al.*, 1973). Viral fevers like those of measles, varicella, or generalized herpes zoster frequently lead to hemorrhagic and necrotic cutaneous lesions. Neurologic lesions, which group meningitis and bacterial and fungal brain abscesses, remain rare. At last, underlying an apparently localized infection, there is a particularly high risk of septicemia.

During the recovery of neutrophil granulocytes, purulent foci with slight inflammatory signs may appear in the regions where the bacteria multiplied, resulting in abscesses of connective tissue, myositis or empyema.

## Septicemias

Fever, systemic symptoms, splenomegaly, existence of a portal of entry, and eventually secondary foci are the main elements which characterize septicemias. When host resistance factors are not weakened, it is not always clinically easy to state with precision when a septicemia develops. During a cancer the problem is even more difficult since systemic symptoms may be considered "normal."

The diagnosis of septicemia may be overlooked owing either to an insufficient number of blood cultures in all febrile cancer patients or to the administration of antibiotics prior to cultures.

They are characterized in these patients, more than in others, by their rapid evolution, the frequency of shock, and the multiplicity of the visceral foci (which are sometimes only proved at necropsy). These are the most usual infectious complications during granulocytopenias and they are all the more frequent when the granulocytopenia is more accentuated (Sickles *et al.*, 1975).

Their confirmation is supported by the rational practice of blood cultures which isolates one or several organisms. These cultures should be repeated if the patient remains febrile despite antibiotic therapy, for they may reveal other bacteria eventually resistant to the applied treatment. In leukemic patients, owing to major granulocytopenia, the absence or the weakness of local inflammatory reactions facilitates the dissemination of organisms in the systemic circulation, which suppress all differences between bacteremia and septicemia. The same is true for all distinctions between saprophytic and pathogenic microorganisms (Loiseau-Marolleau, 1970).

Certain aspects which are particular to the microorganisms and to host resistance shall be precisely stated in Chapter 5.

## BIOLOGIC DIAGNOSIS

Aside from some infections such as varicella, herpes zoster, or measles, the clinical aspect is not sufficiently typical to assure a precise diagnosis of the infection. It is useful to recall the primordial interest of identifying the causal agent for a more precise diagnosis as well as the epidemiology of the infections in order to administer suitable therapy. However, the choice and interpretation of these investigations are sometimes delicate (Table XV).

### General Orientation Tests

Blood cell counts, in the case of granulocytopenia, are not useful in evaluating a bacterial infection. When the leukocytic pool is intact, a leukocytosis with moderate granulocytosis is noted in some solid tumors (in gastrointestinal tract carcinomas particularly) and in Hodgkin's disease (a discrete eosinophilia is also observed) (Bernard, 1967). If, during such malignant diseases complicated with fever, a high leukocytosis of more than $15,000/mm^3$ is observed with a granulocytosis superior to 12,000–13,000, one may consider the possibility of a superinfection such as septicemia from a venous thrombosis origin, a deep suppuration, or bacterial pneumonia. One should not forget that an eosinophilia, sometimes great, may be observed immediately after or in the weeks following irradiation (Ghossein et al., 1975).

It was thought of finding a means for diagnosing bacterial infections by studying the augmentation of phagocytic activity of circulating neutrophil granulocytes by the reduction of tetrazolium nitroblue (NBT). Anderson et al. (1974) observed that in lymphomas with or without fever, but in any event without infection, the reduction of NBT was normal, while it was increased when they were complicated with a bacterial infection. Actually, the positivity of NBT dye test does not appear sufficiently specific, unfortunately, to be used as an important test in bacterial infections (Anner et al., 1975). However, its negativity could be considered as helpful to invalidate the diagnosis of a bacterial infection (Legendre et al., 1976).

The Limulus test brings about gelification of a lysate of ameboid cells prepared from the horseshoe crab (Limulus) in the presence of a few picograms of endotoxin from Gram-negative bacilli. This examination, which is completed in 15 min, gives excellent results in urinary infections (Jorgensen et al., 1973) and in bacterial meningitis caused by Gram-negative bacilli (Nachum et al., 1973), but very inconstant results in the detection of blood endotoxin during septicemias and localized infections (Stumacher et al., 1973). This test may thus have some use in meningitis or urinary infections, in cancer patients.

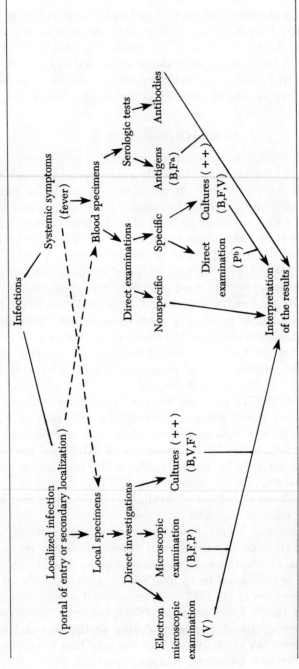

TABLE XV. Laboratory Diagnosis

Note: B = Bacteria; F = Fungi; P = Parasites; V = Virus.
● a *Cryptococcus neoformans.*
●● b *Plasmodium.*

Cytologic specimens taken in lymphadenopathy in cutaneous or subcutaneous lesions, which affirm the presence of malignant cells, rapidly eliminate discussions of an infection.

Finally, the discovery, by leukoconcentration, of circulating malignant cells during febrile malignant lymphomas may have an orientation value for linking the fever to a paraneoplastic mechanism (Hoerni et al., 1970).

### Specific Examinations

**Direct Investigations.** The direct investigations most often used concern bacteria. They should follow certain technical rules for collecting a specimen.

The isolation of the bacteria responsible for the infection is foremost. Specimens should be taken at all possible portals of entry or at the accessible infectious foci, and blood cultures should be done. All specimens should be aseptically collected (to avoid contamination), transported to the laboratory in the best conditions, and cultured aerobically and anaerobically (stools need only to be cultured in aerobiosis.)

Cultures done from specimens with a mixed microbial flora, such as sputum, are significant of an infection if only one or two predominating organisms are isolated. The bacteriologic examination of sputum is difficult owing to buccal contamination at the time of collection; the technique of washing the sputum, or even better direct aspiration (Fig. 4) or the transtrachael puncture (Capped et al., 1973) on the condition that the prothrombin is more than 60% and that there are more than 30,000 platelets/mm$^3$ eliminates this contamination and gives results which are more reliable.

In the event of a septicemia, it is not necessary, except in case of any granulocytopenia, to do more than two to three blood cultures per day, except if an infectious shock complicates the evolution. In this case one or two blood cultures should be done at short intervals prior to antibiotic therapy. In case of severe granulocytopenia, several blood cultures should be done a few hours before antibiotic therapy.

The percentage of positive blood cultures in a series concerning solid tumors and malignant blood diseases varies between 5 and 12% (Lacut et al., 1974; Tapper and Armstrong, 1974). If the efficacy of such an investigation appears weak, its utility is nevertheless evident for screening and treating eventual bacteremias and septicemias. In acute leukemias, the percentage of patients with one or several positive blood cultures is 34% when 1–5 blood cultures were taken, double when 6–10 were taken, but above 10 the percentage of positive cultures does not increase (Loiseau-Marolleau, 1970).

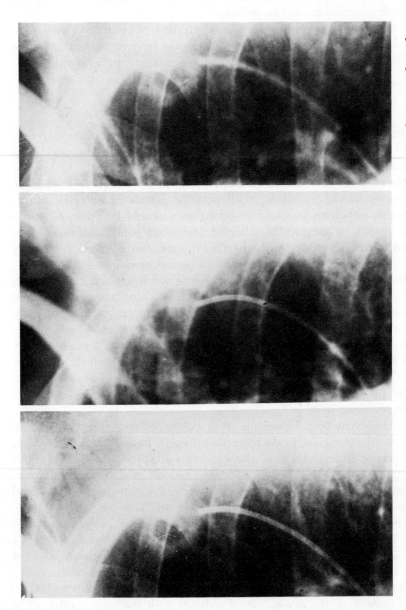

**Fig. 4.** Direct cytologic and bacteriologic aspiration in a axillary abscess by catheter. Displacements depending on respiratory movements.

One should also recall certain rules of interpretation. The results of specimens collected from septic cavities or wounds should be qualitatively and quantitatively interpreted.

Thus an oropharyngeal specimen may include microorganisms considered as commensal (saprophytic *Neisseria,* alpha-hemolytic streptococci) or potentially pathogenic germs (beta-hemolytic streptococci, *Enterobacteriaceae, Pseudomonas*). However, when the latter are only in small number, their responsibility in a focal infection is disputable; on the contrary, in patients with impaired defense these same agents may cause a septicemia or an abscess with septic metastases, even with a minimal portal of entry.

Sputum colony counts, equal or more than $10^6/cm^3$, are considered by some as indicative of a bronchopulmonary infection; others remain sceptical. On the contrary, it is a well-established fact that a bacteriuria equal to or more than $10^5$ is indicative of a urinary infection.

Blood cultures are open to the same discussions. The organisms mainly isolated in cancer patients are *Pseudomonas, Enterobacteriaceae,* and *Staphyloccus aureus.* These bacteria may be considered as either saprophytic or pathogenic and their virulence is affirmed either when they are isolated in blood or are found in large quantities in infectious foci. Generally, *Flavobacterium* is considered as a saprophyte and *Staphylococci epidermidus* as a contaminant, but when they are isolated several times from different blood cultures of the same patient, their pathogenicity is highly probable (see Chapter 5).

Antibiotics and hospitalization select pathogenic organisms, mainly Gram-negative bacilli. Moreover, the portals of entry of infection are most often natural (respiratory, digestive, urinary, cutaneous.)

Hospitalization modifies the resident flora, particularly in the oropharynx, but this notion may be discussed. It had been thought that the pharynx does not harbor many pathogenic Gram-negative bacilli (found in 2% of healthy subjects living outside the hospital environment; Johanson et al., 1969). But with more sophisticated techniques it has recently been demonstrated that *Pseudomonas* and *Enterobacteriaceae* could be found in small numbers in 18% of healthy individuals living outside of a hospital environment (Rosenthal and Tager, 1975).

Classical theories of organism selection in resident flora are evidently pertinent for cancer patients. Thus, it appears that most infections occurring in these patients originate from their resident flora which may be modified by exterior factors, but these factors are generally still poorly defined except for *Pseudomonas aeruginosa* (Schimpff et al., 1973); this has been demonstrated in particular for acute leukemias (Dao, 1971; Schimpff et al., 1972) (see Chapter 3).

Current examinations, done for diagnostic purposes before a presumed infection, may also be used in an attempt to foresee organisms which may, in the future, cause an infection from potential portals of entry. This creates considerable work for the laboratory; nevertheless, in acute nonlymphoid leukemias such research has been done for *Staphylococcus aureus, Enterobacteriaceae,* and *Pseudomonas* (Schimpff *et al.*, 1972). Such an investigation implies the regular repeated collection of specimens from the portals of entry (nose, mouth, hands, feet, armpits, vagina, perianal region, stools, urine), the identification of aerobic pathogenic organisms, and when possible, their serologic typing. It has been demonstrated in acute nonlymphoid leukemias that regular surveillance of the mouth, nose, stools, urine, and axillary regions detected 95% of the organisms responsible for bacterial infections.

Deep infectious foci are not necessarily accompanied by a bacteremia and are difficult to identify. Gallium-citrate scanning aids in their localization when there is a severe granulocytipenia, but this isotopic product is also retained by the cancerous tissue, thus giving false positive results (Littenberg *et al.*, 1973; Oster *et al.*, 1975). It is probably more interesting to label granulocytes: for example, these cells can phagocytose particles labeled with technetium-99m and then, after this labeling, can be reinjected in subjects by autotransfusion. Such an investigation has given good results in animal experiments as well as promising preliminary data in humans (Armengaud *et al.*, 1976). It is probably possible to use allogeneic labeled granulocytes in patients with severe granulocytopenia.

The isolation of a virus is not proof of its responsibility in an infection. The proof is assured only by the demonstration of an associated signifying increase in antibody titer.

The signification of an isolation of *Candida* in sputum, mouth, or stools is open to the same type of discussion. The reality of a buccal or digestive candidiasis is easier to determine, whereas that of a pulmonary mycosis is much more delicate and is sometimes established only by a lung biopsy (an examination which cannot always be done). The same remarks may be made for pneumocystosis.

The diagnostic difficulties raised by multiple pulmonary abnormalities, usually described as "interstitial" pneumonias, underlie the value of pulmonary biopsy. Open lung biopsies give the best results: 95 lung biopsy procedures in 78 immunocompromised patients (among them there were 57 cancer patients) yielded valuable diagnoses in 35% of the needle aspirates, 46% of the cutting needle biopsies, and 65% of the open thoracotomies (Greenman *et al.*, 1975). There is no absolute contraindication to these procedures. Nevertheless, it is sometimes necessary to correct coagulation deficiency: a prothrombin time of less than 60%

significantly increases hemorrhagic complications. A moderate isolated thrombocytopenia does not increase hemorrhagic hazards, but it is necessary to give thrombocyte transfusions before and immediately after surgical intervention if thrombocytopenia is less than 100,000/mm$^3$. In patients with hematologic neoplasms, different specimens obtained by such pulmonary biopsies show either infectious isolated or multiple lesions (pneumocystosis, fungal infection, bacterial infection, tuberculosis, virosis, particularly cytomegalovirosis), cancerous especially lymphomatous lesions, or nonspecific inflammatory manifestations (Table XVI; Greenman et al., 1975; Marty et al., 1975; Abdallah et al., 1976; Iyer et al., 1976; Neiman et al., 1976). These procedures improve the prognosis of these otherwise undiagnosable interstitial pneumonias since they sometimes given an early diagnosis and thus allow an appropriate treatment (Greenman et al., 1975).

Finally, besides microorganism isolation, fruitful researches have been performed over the last few years to detect some bacterial antigens (meningococcus, pneumococcus, Haemophilus influenzae) by counterimmunoelectrophoresis or latex-particle agglutination. These bacterial antigens may be identified either in cerebrospinal fluid in meningitis caused by the aforementioned microorganisms (Coonrod and Rytel, 1972; Whittle et al., 1974) or in blood, or better in sputum in Pneumococcus pneumonias (Dorff et al., 1971; Tugwell and Greenwood, 1974). Among fungi, Cryptococcus neoformans alone is the one whose antigens can be identified in serum or cerebrospinal fluid (Bloomfield et al., 1963; Bindschadler and Bennett, 1968). These procedures are useful for diagnosis and treatment, especially for cancer patients in whom microorganisms are sometimes scarce. Other bacterial or fungal antigens must be searched for in the same way.

**Serologic Tests.** Cancer patients retain the possibility of synthesizing antibodies for a long time; thus serologic reactions are useful. Serologic studies done in patients with solid tumors or blood malignancies after

TABLE XVI.  Distribution of Pulmonary Disease Diagnosed by Lung Biopsy in Patients with Hematologic Neoplasms[a]

| Underlying Neoplasm | Pulmonary Disease | | | | |
| --- | --- | --- | --- | --- | --- |
| | Neoplastic Lesion | Specific Infection | Nonspecific Inflammation | No Diagnosis | Total |
| Hodgkin's disease | 17 | 4 | 2 | 2 | 25 |
| Other lymphoma | 5 | 5 | 2 | 7 | 19 |
| Leukemia | 0 | 4 | 4 | 3 | 11 |
| Total | 22 | 13 | 8 | 12 | 55 |

[a] From Greenman et al. (1975).

positive blood cultures with Gram-negative bacilli (mainly *Escherichia coli* and *Klebsiella*) showed that more than half of the patients developed specific antibodies directed against the somatic O antigens for the corresponding microorganisms: 69.7% during solid tumors and 44% during malignant blood diseases (Surgalla *et al.*, 1975). Infections caused by cytomegalovirus have been particularly studied during hematologic neoplasms. Bussel *et al.* (1975) report 33 cases and observe a significant increase in antibody titer in 31 of them.

Among many serologic tests there is one which is particular to staphylococcemia: it is possible to search for serum antibodies against cell-wall teichoic acids of *Staphylococcus aureus* by gel diffusion or counterimmunoelectrophoresis (Tuazon and Sheagren, 1976). This test is positive after 8–15 days. Its specificity and its rapidity (40 min for the counterimmunoelectrophoresis) seem especially useful in staphylococcemias developing in immunocompromised hosts.

The interpretation of serodiagnosis here, as elsewhere, follows a number of classic rules and depends on qualitative, quantitative, and evolutive data.

The specificity of serologic reactions is limited. Different microorganisms have certain antigens in common and give cross-reactions: for example, *Salmonella paratyphi* B and *Salmonella typhimurium* have a part of their O antigen in common, as well as *Salmonella typhi* and *Salmonella enteritidis*. In addition, preexisting antibody titers may arise because of pathologic conditions which are not reinfections caused by corresponding organisms.

The titer of an antigen-antibody reaction must be sufficiently high to have a pathologic value. An antistreptolysin O titer of 240 or greater in a school-age patient or 120 or greater in a preschool-age or adult patient is suggestive of a recent group A beta-hemolytic streptococcal infection. However, isolated quantitative criteria are often insufficient; this again points out the value of acute and convalescent series.

A recent infection causes antibody production in a delay of 8–15 days with a rapid augmentation of their titer. They persist in the host in a variable manner. Certain remain only a few weeks (anti-O antibodies of typhoid and paratyphoid fevers, complement fixation test in viral diseases), while other remain, sometimes at high titers, for months, or even years (antibodies which inhibit hemagglutination in rubella, antitoxoplasmosis antibodies). A serodiagnosis is generally positive when there is a frank augmentation in antibody titer, equal or superior to four dilutions in two blood samples, one realized at the beginning of the disease and the second one 15 days later. The rule of two serologic examinations done at 15-day intervals is most valuable.

Thus it is useful to have a baseline antibody titer for a patient. This implies that blood samples must be systematically taken for all patients before any signs of infection exist. One cannot search for any and al! antibodies for each patient, but the serum could be frozen until needed. Then, if and when an infection develops, a second blood sample could be taken and the two specimens could be simultaneously tested to compare the antibody titers. The laboratory cannot stock frozen blood samples for all patients, but perhaps it can for those with high infectious risks, such as hematologic malignancies, at least for acute leukemias.

These serologic reactions, perhaps more in cancer patients than in other patients, run the risk of being erroneously interpreted, even when they have been done correctly.

False positive Weil-Fely serologic reactions are frequent in patients vaccinated against typhoid fevers, but have also been noted during malignant blood diseases, particularly in dysglobulinemia, or during superinfected colon cancer, even if no evidence of an associated typhoid fever exists (Bastin and Frottier, 1969). The proof of toxoplasmosis rests practically on serology alone and its interpretation follows classical rules, but positive results do not necessarily signify a current parasitosis (see Chapter 8).

On the other hand, there are reactions which give false negative results (technical laboratory errors being excluded). These reactions may be linked to the character of the infection which is too localized, or to the nature of the antigen (not all cases of infectious mononucleosis give a positive Paul–Bunnell test), or to an immunosuppression which is too great. For systemic candidiasis (Rosner et al., 1971) and aspergillosis (Meyer et al., 1973) occurring during cancers, serologic data are not precise enough to confirm a difficult diagnosis. However, Schaefer et al. (1976) observed seven serologic conversions (negative to positive) with a specific Aspergillus fumigatus immunodiffusion test performed twice a week in 10 patients with acute nonlymphoid leukemia and actual aspergillosis. Pneumocystosis is inconstantly accompanied by specific antibodies: an indirect immunofluorescence test gives only 40 to 50% of positive results in patients with Pneumocystis pneumonia (Walzer et al., 1974; Arnaud et al., 1976).

These considerations about the general clinical and biological characteristics of infections during cancer give a better diagnostic approach, but have variable difficulties. Sometimes the infection, especially when it is bacterial, is so severe in these patients that after a few biological examinations it is necessary to undertake an antibiotic association which will hopefully be efficacious. This therapy may be revised later by the results of the in vitro sensitivity tests. These data will be developed in Chapters 5–8 depending on the nature of the responsible pathogenic agents.

# 2

# Diagnosis and
# Clinical Manifestations

CHAPTER 5

# Bacterial Infections

Bacterial infections in solid tumors are favored by special local conditions (stenosis, obstruction, and ulceration) and develop at rather advanced stages of malignancy. The most severe infections appear during malignant blood diseases, particularly in acute leukemias. Severe granulocytopenias, which are linked to cancer but are also frequently owing to anticancer chemotherapy, markedly increase the incidence and gravity of bacterial infections.

These bacterial infections are the most current and most severe of all infections, and are the main cause of mortality from infectious origin, coming before hemorrhagic or thromboembolic accidents and cancer itself in the causes of death in cancer patients (see Chapter 11).

The responsible microorganisms are mainly represented by the Gram-negative bacilli. The *Enterobacteriaceae* and the obligate aerobic bacteria are the microorganisms most often encountered, regardless of the anatomic site of infection, but any type of bacteria may actually be involved.

The epidemiology of these bacterial infections and the factors which favor them have been discussed in Chapters 1–3.

Out of 2988 blood cultures done in febrile cancer patients, Sinkovics and Smith (1969) found 364 positive cultures: about 70% of the Gram-negative bacilli are represented by *Escherichia coli, Pseudomonas, Klebsiella, Serrattia, Enterobacter,* and *Proteus* (Table XVII). In a study on myeloma, Meyers *et al.* (1972) confirm the high incidence of Gram-negative bacilli, which are responsible for three-quarters of the infections observed, regardless of their type.

These Gram-negative bacterial infections are grave; they develop not only in compromised patients, but, in addition, are characterized by their resistance to antibiotics (these microorganisms readily acquire transferable multiple resistances). We shall recall that these acquired bacterial resistances to one or several antibiotics (polymyxin and rifampin appear, for the moment, excluded) result from simple enzymatic reactions coded by fragments of extrachromosomic DNA autosomes called plasmids, also called the R factor or RTF (resistance transfer factor); they include, in addition to genetic determinants, which are

TABLE XVII.   Microorganisms Isolated by Blood Cultures from Cancer Patients[a,b]

| | | |
|---|---:|---:|
| Gram-negative bacilli | | 263 |
|    *E. coli* | 101 | |
|    *Klebsiella, Serratia, Enterobacter* | 78 | |
|    *Proteus* | 20 | |
|    *Salmonella* | 4 | |
|    *Pseudomonas* | 57 | |
|    Miscellaneous | 3 | |
| Gram-positive cocci | | 70 |
|    *Streptococcus* | 39 | |
|    *Diplococcus pneumoniae* | 10 | |
|    *Staphylococcus aureus* | 21 | |
| Gram-positive bacilli | | 10 |
| Obligate anaerobic agents (*Bacteroides, Clostridium*) | | 12 |
| Fungi (*Candida*) | | 9 |
|    Total | | 364 |

[a] Patients with more than one positive blood culture for the same agent and those with a septicemia due to two microorganisms are included in this series.

[b] From Sinkovics and Smith (1969), 1966–1968; M.D. Anderson Hospital, Houston, Texas.

responsible for the resistance to a particular antibiotic, elements which permit their transfer. In the Gram-negative bacilli they are readily transmissible by conjugation from one bacterium to another. These bacteria may belong to different families or groups. Presently 60–70% of bacteria carry resistance plasmids.

According to their portal of entry and their virulence, these microorganisms cause infections which cover all aspects of bacterial pathology. It is, however, useful to distinguish the usual aspects of infections during solid tumors from particular aspects of those during malignant blood diseases and severe granulocytopenias.

The general diagnostic problems of bacterial infections have been discussed in Chapter 4. The main clinical features found will be discussed here: certain aspects of localized infections (pneumonias, perirectal and perianal abscesses, meningitis) will be considered first because of their singularity, frequency, and gravity. Septicemias, complications particularly common in cancer patients, will then be analyzed. Finally, there will be a discussion on mycobacterial infections.

## LOCALIZED INFECTIONS

### Bronchopulmonary Infections

These complications appear either as a result of local pulmonary alteration, for example, a neoplastic bronchial stenosis (see Chapter 4) or in lung parenchyma without cancer.

In a series by Klastersky *et al.*, (1971), 37 cancers, complicated by batcerial pneumonias, included 29 solid tumors (12 of which were bronchogenic carcinomas or pulmonary metastasis). In only seven cases the number of granulocytes was low (between 500 and 2600/mm$^3$). *Klebsiella pneumoniae* and *Pseudomonas aeruginosa* were the microorganisms most often found (Table XVIII). Radiologically, pneumonic obstruction was rare, and the most common lesions were basal bronchopneumonias (16 unilateral and 10 bilateral). The 5 complicated cases of empyema were fatal; out of the 6 septicemias 5 were fatal. With two exceptions, all these infections were probably hospital-acquired infections. Those which developed in the first 6 days of admission had a lower mortality rate (40%) than those which developed belatedly (70%). The overall mortality was 62% and the mean survival time of patients with these fatal infectious was 9.2 days. This survival time was shorter for pneumonias caused by *Klebsiella* (5.5 days) than for pneumonias caused by other bacteria. The mortality of these pulmonary infections in solid tumors was 58%; this rate approached the one found in acute leukemias and was explained by the high proportion of generalized cancers (22 out of 29 cases).

Bacterial pneumonias are also very common but have a particular aspect in acute leukemias. In these patients they may be associated with other microorganisms which colonize the lung; fungi (Sickles *et al.*, 1973), *Pneumocystis carinii* (Goodell *et al.*, 1970), and cytomegalovirus (Cangir *et al.*, 1967). These pneumonias, acquired in the hospital and caused by one or two organisms, are mainly due to Gram-negative bacilli (*Pseudomonas aeruginosa, Klebsiella, E. coli*), and more rarely to staphylococci or pneumococci (Table XIX). These microorganisms colonize the upper respiratory tract and are the source of infection. Fever is constant, dyspnea is very frequent, while coughing and expectoration are found in less than two-thirds of the cases. These pneumonias have a tendency to be diffuse (especially those caused by *Klebsiella*) and to be bilateral with a predominance of basal lesions, simulating congestive heart failure, but in these cases the central venous pressure remains low (lower than 10 cm of water), at least in the beginning (Iannini *et al.*, 1974). These pneumonias, in particular those caused by *Pseudomonas aeruginosa*, include vasculitis, necrotic foci, and microabscesses, but they seldom cause large abscesses (Sickles *et al.*, 1973). They are very severe infections, fatal in two-thirds of the cases. The associated severe granulocytopenia and septicemia worsen the prognosis: 100% of the pneumonias caused by *Pseudomonas aeruginosa*, complicated by a septicemia,

TABLE XVIII.  Pulmonary Infections due to Gram-Negative Bacilli in Cancer Patients[a]

| Microorganisms | Number of isolated Bacteria | Clinical Picture | | | | | |
|---|---|---|---|---|---|---|---|
| | | Fever | Dyspnea | Purulent Sputum | Radiologic Abnormalities | Pleuritis Purulent | Septicemia |
| Klebsiella[b] | 16 | 14 | 3 | 11 | 16 | 1 | 3 |
| Proteus mirabilis | 3 | 3 | 1 | 3 | 3 | 3 | 0 |
| E. coli | 3 | 3 | 1 | 2 | 3 | 1 | 2 |
| Pseudomonas aeruginosa | 15 | 15 | 8 | 14 | 3 | 0 | 1 |
| Total[b] | 37 | 35 | 13 | 30 | 31 | 5 | 6 |

[a] From Klastersky et al. (1971), Jules-Bordet Institute, Brussels.
[b] Plus one enterobacteria.

are lethal (Pennington *et al.*, 1973); out of 36 cases collected in this latter series there were 18 acute leukemias, 2 chronic myeloid leukemias, 1 chronic lymphoid leukemia, and 7 solid tumors.

*Nocardia asteroides* is an opportunistic agent which is sometimes responsible for pulmonary manifestations in cancer, renal-transplanted (Cohen *et al.*, 1971), and cardiac-transplanted patients (Krick *et al.*, 1975). Sometimes these microorganisms are found only at the commensal state, other times they cause bronchopneumonic lesions, necrotizing pneumonia, pulmonary abscess, and sometimes skin, liver, or brain abscesses (Young *et al.*, 1971). These filamentous aerobic bacteria belong to the *Actinomycetaceae* family, grow slowly, and have a characteristic morphology in sputum smears. They are not organisms of superinfection. Out of 13 patients (series of Young *et al.*, 1971) who developed nocardiosis, 8 had a lymphoma (5 of which were Hodgkin's disease). These microorganisms are sensitive to sulfonamides, which can be effective in spite of the underlying malignancy. Thus, in the same series, 2 patients with Hodgkin's disease were cured of their nocardic pulmonary abscess, while 11 others died of either that infection, a septicemia (caused by Gram-negative bacilli, or *Staphyloccocus aureus*), or a hemorrhage.

Finally, *Mycoplasma pneumoniae* (microorganisms which belong to

TABLE XIX.   Pneumonias in Patients with Acute Leukemia: Microorganisms Isolated in 37 Patients[a]

| Microorganisms | Site of Isolation | | | Total[b] |
| --- | --- | --- | --- | --- |
| | Sputum | Blood | Lung (postmortem) | |
| P. aeruginosa | 1 | 8 | 5 | 9 |
| Other *Pseudomonas* | 0 | 1 | 2 | 3 |
| Klebsiella | 2 | 4 | 5 | 7 |
| Enterobacter | 0 | 2 | 3 | 4 |
| E. coli | 0 | 4 | 2 | 5 |
| Staph. aureus | 2 | 0 | 2 | 3 |
| D. pneumoniae | 0 | 2 | 0 | 2 |
| Streptococcus D | 2 | 2 | 1 | 5 |
| H. influenzae | 1 | 0 | 0 | 1 |
| Candida | 1 | 6 | 8 | 12 |
| Aspergillus | 0 | 0 | 1 | 1 |
| Total | 9 | 29 | 29 | 52[c] |

[a] From Sickles *et al.* (1973), Cancer Research Center, Baltimore, Maryland.
[b] Several microorganisms were isolated from different sites.
[c] Two microorganisms were isolated for 15 pneumonias.

the class of mollicutes, different from bacteria or viruses), an agent of primary atypical pneumonia, does not seem to be particularly more responsible for pathologic manifestations in cancer patients than in other patients. However, obstructive disease or diffuse reticulonodular infiltrations have been attributed to this microorganisms during Hodgkin's disease (Putman et al., 1975). Pulmonary infiltrations seem to result from an immunologic reaction and develop more readily as the immunologic reactions of the patient are conserved (Foy et al., 1973). These infections respond to tetracycline or erythromycin.

## Perianal and Perirectal Abscesses

These suppurating complications generally develop only when a severe granulocytopenia (less than 500/mm$^3$) exists; they are mainly seen in acute leukemias (23 out of 25 times in the Schimpff et al. series, 1972), especially the nonlymphoid type (Table IV). Their pathogenesis is not clear. Mucous-membrane ulcerations might be favored by the action of muramidase, abundantly secreted by malignant cells in acute monocytic and myelomonocytic leukemias; moreover, specific submucous infiltrations (Fig. 5), common in acute monocytic leukemia, could also play a role in the appearance of fissures and abscesses. In this series, 14 patients already had hemorrhoids and 20 had digestive disorders: diarrhea, constipation, or digestive hemorrhages. Finally, the thermometer could have played a role, either by causing an ulceration or by introducing pathogenic microorganisms.

Varying in size from 1 to 8 cm, these abscesses are very painful, seldom fluctuant, and are surrounded by inflammatory and indurated tissues. Their puncture gives a cloudy liquid with few granulocytes. The culture of these abscesses shows a mixed flora with a predominance of Pseudomonas, but anaerobic organisms are also present. In 15 cases, these lesions were complicated by septicemia; 12 of these septicemias were caused by Pseudomonas aeruginosa and 12 had a fatal evolution.

The management of these abscesses primarily consists of regulating the digestive passage, a low-fiber diet, or local wet compresses, and administering an antibiotic therapy which may later be modified by the results of in vitro sensitivity tests. In the evolutive phase of blood disease, the best local therapy seems to be radiotherapy (300–400 rads in 1–3 days to the lesion). If the induration persists or reappears, radiotherapy may be repeated one week later. Drainage should be limited to a simple incision and done only when there is a fluctuation of the abscess. More complex surgery, incision and drainage, sphincterotomy, fissurectomy, hemorrhoid ablation (Sehdev et al., 1973), even a

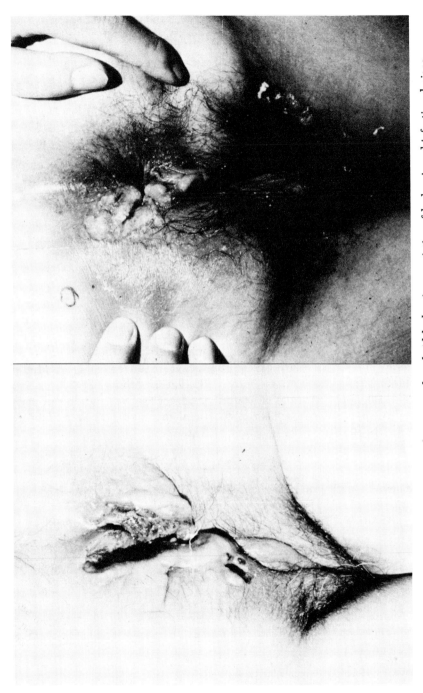

**Fig. 5** Anal lesions in two patients with acute nonlymphoid leukemia: association of leukemic and infectious lesions.

diverting colostomy (Schimpff *et al.*, 1972), should be considered only in patients who have a sufficient number of granulocytes and platelets and are in remission.

## Meningitis

Bacterial meningitis develops in leukemias, dysglobulinemias, and lymphomas but is rare considering the frequency of infections in these diseases: 9 cases (1.25%) out of 717 malignant blood diseases in our experience (Lacut *et al.*, 1974).

In chronic leukemias, mainly lymphoid, as well as in dysglobuline-mias, the responsible organisms are above all the pyogenic bacteria, such as *Pneumococcus* and *Pseudomonas*. In acute leukemias, although Gram-negative bacilli predominate, *Listeria monocytogenes* is often found. Finally in lymphomas, *Listeria* is the most often isolated etiologic agent (Table XX).

The clinical aspects of these meningitides are generally typical but sometimes may be overlooked owing to meningeal hemorrhage (Lacut *et al.*, 1974) or leukemic meningitis (Durand *et al.*, 1976). Thus it is extremely important to culture all cerebrospinal fluids collected during routine examination in meningeal hemorrhage, leukemic meningitis (Fig.6), or intrathecal anticancer treatment. If the slightest doubt of bacterial meningitis exists, an appropriate, generalized, and intrathecal antibiotic therapy should be started. Similar to other infections, men-ingitis also appears at an advanced stage of cancer and has a high mortality rate; out of 29 cases of bacterial meningitis 14 were fatal, 9 occurred in 10 patients with leukemia (Table XXI).

## SEPTICEMIAS

Their portal of entry has been discussed in Chapters 3 and 4.

TABLE XX.   Distribution of Listeriosis According to the Type of Cancer

| Cancer | Louria *et al.* (1967) | Durand *et al.* (1976)[a] |
|---|---|---|
| Acute leukemia | 3 | 7 |
| Chronic leukemia | 3 | 6 |
| Hodgkin's disease | 8 | 7 |
| Non-Hodgkin's lymphoma | 3 | 4 |
| Solid tumor | 1 | 0 |
| Total | 18 | 24 |

[a] Review including only meningitis in blood malignancies.

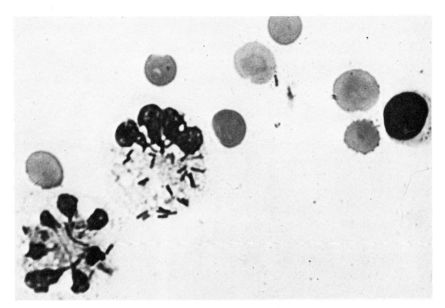

**Fig. 6.** Meningeal listeriosis. Cerebrospinal fluid of a patient with acute lymphoid leukemia and lymphoblastic meningitis. In the cytoplasm of two very altered granulocytes there are a number of rods with prolonged pseudofilamentous forms of *Listeria*.

In cancer patients septicemias caused by Gram-negative bacilli are readily complicated by severe endotoxin shock accompanied by hypotension or collapse, reduction of blood volume, decrease of cardiac output, slowing down of circulation, peripheral vasoconstriction, oliguria, hyperlacticacidemia, tendency toward acidosis, and the possibility of disseminated intravascular coagulation. Although Gram-negative septicemias are generally accompanied by fever, it is useful to note that some of them cause an immediate hypothermia, even without any associated collapse.

Septicemias caused by Gram-positive microorganisms cause fewer hemodynamic problems, and are generally characterized by a normal cardiac output, no increased peripheral resistances, normal circulation, and maintenance of cardiac and urine output. If acute hypotension exists, it appears to be due to peripheral vasodilatation.

The obligate anaerobes, excluding *Clostridium perfringens,* do not give any particular clinical signs. It is presently recognized that *Clostridium* does not necessarily provoke hemolysis, collapse, and oligoanuria by interstitial tubular renal disease.

The clinical evolution depends on multiple factors, the most important

TABLE XXI. Prognosis of Bacterial Meningitis in Patients with Blood Malignancies[a]

| Blood Malignancies | Number of Cases of Meningitis | Evolution of Meningitis | | Further Evolution of Patients Recovering from Meningitis |
|---|---|---|---|---|
| | | Death | Recovery | |
| Malignant lymphomas | 10 | 2 | 8 | 1 death from bronchopneumonia<br>1 death from Hodgkin's disease and multiple infections |
| Acute leukemias | 10 | 9 | 1 | 1 death from *Candida* septicemia |
| Chronic leukemias | 6 | 3 | 3 | 2 deaths from other infections<br>1 death from another cancer |
| Myelomas | 3 | 0 | 3 | 1 death from myeloma |
| Total | 29 | 14 | 15 | |

[a] From Lacut *et al.* (1974).

of which depends on the underlying malignancy, the state of the bone marrow, and the importance of the granulocytopenia. Septicemias are much more severe in acute leukemias resistant to chemotherapy than in newly diagnosed acute leukemias and hypoplasias induced by chemotherapy (Atkinson *et al.*, 1974). Finally, prognosis of Gram-positive septicemias seems to be better than the prognosis of Gram-negative septicemias (Atkinsin *et al.*, 1974).

Most septicemias are caused by only 1 organism, but it is not rare to isolate 2 or even 3 organisms in different blood cultures from the same patient. In 52 speticemias caused by *Pseudomonas*, a second microorganism was isolated in 9 cases (Tapper and Armstrong, 1974); 2 and sometimes 3 bacteria have successively been isolated in 11 out of 50 leukemia cases complicated by septicemia (Loiseau-Marolleau, 1970).

### Septicemias Caused by Gram-Negative Bacilli

All Gram-negative bacilli may cause septicemias, especially *E. coli* and *Klebsiella*, but those caused by *Pseudomonas* have been studied the most. For Fishman and Armstrong (1972) they represent 25% of the septicemias caused by Gram-negative bacilli. Since the important series of Sinkovics and Smith (1969) (Table XVII), Schimpff *et al.* (1973) have shown that among the organisms responsible for 93 septicemias in cancer patients, *Pseudomonas aeruginosa* was responsible 26 times, *Klebsiella* 11 times, and *E. coli* 8 times.

Most septicemias caused by *Pseudomonas* are hospital-acquired infections: out of 52 observed cases, 48 developed during hospitalization (Tapper and Armstrong, 1974). Patients colonized with this organism develop septicemias more frequently if they suffer from leukemia than lymphomas, brain tumors, or a cancer with metastasis (Schimpff *et al.*, 1973).

In their origin granulocytopenia is an essential factor. Infections caused by *Pseudomonas* do not develop in patients having more than 1000 circulating granulocytes, while 44% of patients carrying this microorganism develop a septicemia when the number of granulocytes falls below 1000 per cubic millimeter (Schimpff *et al.*, 1973).

Out of 21 septicemias caused by *Pseudomonas* in cancer patients (Table XXII), Forkner *et al.* (1958) noted 20 deaths between 1 to 10 days, with a mean survival time of 4.3 days starting from the first signs of infection. In this series, aside from lung localizations, one observes the frequency of meningeal disorders (5 cases developing in leukemias, 3 of which were acute leukemias), jaundice (11/21), and skin lesions (9/21). The latter may present four main aspects: common ecthyma

TABLE XXII.   Distribution of Septicemias due to Pseudomonas According to the Type of Cancer

| Cancers | Centers and References | | | |
|---|---|---|---|---|
| | Cancer Center, Bethesda (Forkner et al., 1958) | Memorial Hospital, New York (Fishman and Armstrong, 1972) | Cancer Center, Baltimore (Schimpff et al., 1973) | Memorial Hospital, New York (Tapper and Armstrong, 1974) |
| Acute leukemia | | | | |
| lymphoid | 10 | 11 | 1 | 22 |
| nonlymphoid | 3 | | 15 | |
| Chronic leukemia | 3 | 2 | 0 | 4 |
| Malignant lymphoma | | | | |
| Hodgkin's | 2 | 1 | 3 | 10 |
| non-Hodgkin's | | 16 | 4 | |
| Solid tumor | 3 | 19 | 3 | 14 |
| Total | 21 | 49 | 26 | 50 |

gangrenosum (Fig. 7), vesicles which tend to group in clumps and either completely heal or evolve toward ecthyma, cellulitis with hemorrhagic and necrotic evolution, and maculopapular lesions or nodules.

Fishman and Armstrong (1972) reported 50 septicemias caused by *Pseudomonas* in 46 cancer patients. In order of frequency the portals of entry were cutaneous (30%), urinary (26%), pulmonary (22%), and perineal (12%). The importance of the hemodynamic consequences was emphasized: in 70% of the cases there was hypotension or collapse. Thirty-nine patients (78%) succumbed to septicemia caused by *Pseudomonas* (100% mortality in lymphomas; 72% in leukemias, 58% in other patients); 21 among them (42%) died in 24 hr or less after an irreversible infectious shock. Tapper and Armstrong (1974) indicated that the most frequent portals of entry (60%) were pulmonary and urinary and also noted a mortality of 69% despite diagnostic progress and rapid appropriate antibiotic treatment. In nonlymphoid acute leukemia, the infectious foci most often associated with septicemia are pulmonary and anorectal (Schimpff *et al.*, 1973), whereas in other cancers they are pulmonary and urinary (Fig. 8).

*Serratia*, another multiresistant bacteria of the opportunistic flora, causes localized infections (particularly urinary disorders) rather than septicemias (10 septicemias in a series of 32 patients of Bodey *et al.*, 1970) (Table XXIII). These septicemias have no particular clinical signs, but develop readily after important surgical interventions and after urinary-tract catheterization.

*Salmonella*, in addition to being the bacteria responsible for typhoid and paratyphoid fevers, mainly cause gastroenteritis. *Salmonella* may become more virulent in compromised hosts, causing septicemias, and/or localized infections (pneumonia, empyema, cholecystitis, appendicitis, peritonitis, salpingitis, urinary or osteoarticular infections, and meningitis). These bacteria are seldom responsible for infections in cancer patients (Table XXIII), but their frequency is higher in cancer patients than in others (Sinkovics and Smith, 1969). In our experience, we have observed 10 cases of salmonellosis in cancer patients (only in patients with blood malignancy). Generally, their epidemiology has not been studied.

In a series of 100 cases of salmonellosis collected over 13 years and excluding typhoid fever, Wolfe *et al.* (1971) reported gastroenteritis (37%), focal infections (16%), and carriers (12%). In addition there were 35 septicemias: two-thirds were due to *Salmonella typhimurium* and 32 concerned cancer patients. Three-quarters of these septicemias developed in patients with leukemia or malignant lymphoma.

Sometimes other Gram-negative bacilli may be incrimated. *Aero-*

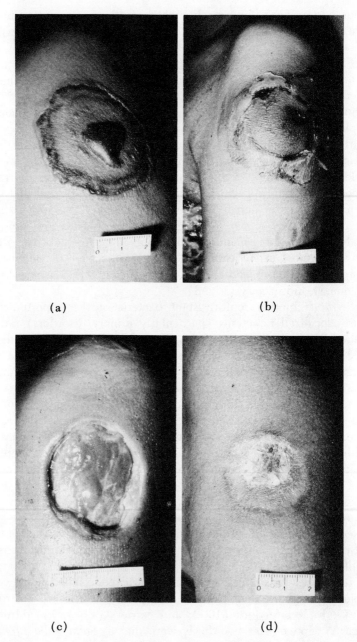

(a)                              (b)

(c)                              (d)

**Fig. 7.** Evolution of an ecthyma gangrenosum due to *Pseudomonas aeruginosa* in the left deltoid area in a 33-year-old woman suffering advanced breast cancer: (*a*) October 21; (*b*) October 28; (*c*) November 11; (*d*) December 20.

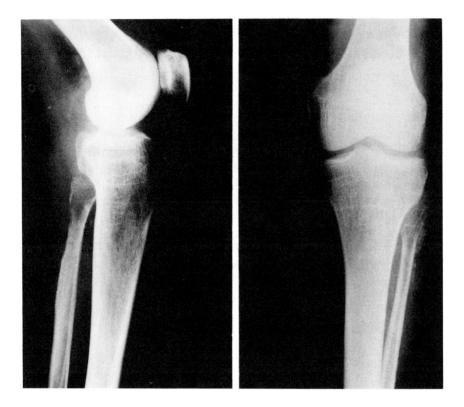

**Fig. 8.** Pseudomonas osteitis in a patient with multiple myeloma following a septicemia.

*monas* are microorganisms which are usually present in water, earth, and diverse food products. They are a source of infection in some animals, like fish and amphibians. They are rarely involved in human pathology but they are pathogenic mainly in cirrhotic or cancer patients. Some septicemias caused by *Aeromonas hydrophila* have been reported in cancer patients, particularly in hematologic neoplasms (Brisou *et al.*, 1975; Soussy *et al.*, 1975). In some septicemias developing in leukemic patients, *Aeromonas hydrophila* has also been isolated from cutaneous lesions, mainly ecthyma gangrenosum (Dean and Post, 1967; Shilkin *et al.*, 1968; Ketover *et al.*, 1973). *Yersinia enterocoliticia*, which is usually responsible for enterocolitis, acute syndromes of the right iliac fossa, and erythema nodosum, may cause septicemias mainly in compromised hosts. One such case has been reported in a chronic lymphoid leukemia (Mollaret *et al.*, 1971). Finally, *Haemophilus aphrophilus* was isolated from eight blood cultures in patients with acute myeloid leukemia who presented a clinical picture of bacterial endocarditis (Enck and Bennett, 1976).

## Septicemias Caused by Gram-Positive Microorganisms

These agents are definitely less important as causes of septicemias (Sinkovics and Smith, 1969; Gaya et al., 1973).

The staphylococci which were isolated during septicemias were mainly *Staphylococcus aureus*, while *Staphylococcus epidermididis* is seldom mentioned or reported as being exceptional (Loiseau-Marolleau, 1970). To consider *Staphylococcus epidermididis* isolated once in one blood culture as being a contaminant is logical, but when it is isolated from several blood cultures in the same patient, its pathogenicity becomes highly probable. Septicemias caused by *Staphylococcus epidermididis* remain more rare in cancer patients than in patients with artificial cardiac valves, pacemakers, or in drug addicts (Worms, 1969).

Beta-hemolytic group A *Streptococcus*, a bacteria seldom isolated in septicemias of cancer patients, seems to be found more frequently in solid tumors than in other malignancies (Table XXIV). These septicemias are accompanied by high white blood cell counts (more than 10,000 leukocytes) in half of the observations. They are consequences of surgery in 24% of the cases and have a mortality rate of 21% when the diagnosis is made during the lifetime of the patient. If one corrects the percentage by adding the cases in which blood cultures are positive postmortem (Henkel et al., 1970), the mortality rate is 45%.

Other streptococci may cause septicemias. Group B *Streptococcus* has recently been signaled as the etiologic agent of septicemias in malignant blood diseases (Lerner et al., 1975). This bacteria, a frequent host of the female genital tract, is more often responsible for neonatal infections.

*Pneumococci* normally colonize the respiratory tract. In everyday infectious pathology it is responsible for otitis and lung infections. In oncology its responsibility in septicemias is limited: 10 blood cultures were positive for this bacteria out of 364 positive blood cultures (Sinkovics and Smith, 1969). Sixty observations of septicemias caused by pneumococci (Table XXIV) have been collected from 1955 to 1971 in a cancer center (Folland et al., 1974): malignant blood disease occurred in half of the patients even though the percentage of admissions in that hospital for leukemias, lymphomas, and myelomas was only 6% during that time interval. Among the solid tumors, lung cancer is found only four times. However, the onset of septicemia is pulmonary in two-thirds of the cases and pneumococci have been isolated in the

TABLE XXIII.  Distribution of Infections due to Other Gram-Negative Bacilli
According to the Type of Cancer

| | Centers and References | | |
| | Serratia | Salmonella | |
| Cancers | M.D. Anderson Hospital, Houston (Bodey *et al.*, 1970) | M.D. Anderson Hospital, Houston (Sinkovics and Smith, 1969) | Memorial Hospital, New York (Wolfe *et al.*, 1971) |
|---|---|---|---|
| Leukemias | 9 | 11 | 21 |
| Malignant lymphomas | 0 | 5 | 25 |
| Urogenital cancers | 14 | 9 | 15 |
| Gastrointestinal cancers | 7 | 2 | 9 |
| Other cancers | 2 | 6 | 16 |
| Total | 32 | 33 | 86 |

TABLE XXIV.    Distribution of Bacteremias due to Gram-Positive Cocci
According to the Type of Cancer

| Cancers | Memorial Hospital, New York | |
|---|---|---|
| | Henkel et al. (1970) | Folland et al. (1974) |
| | Beta-hemolytic Group A Streptococcus | Pneumococcus |
| Acute leukemias | 5 | 8 |
| Chronic leukemias | 1 | 7 |
| Malignant lymphomas | 9 | 14 |
| Gastrointestinal cancers | 9 | 12 |
| Breast cancers | 6 | 2 |
| Lung cancers | 2 | 4 |
| Other cancers | 14 | 12 |
| Total | 46 | 59 |

sputum in nearly half of the cases analyzed during pneumonias. Five times it was responsible for a purulent meningitis. Most of the patients were febrile, but 10 did not have fever at the time the bacteria were isolated although they did have an infectious foci. In spite of the efficacy of antibiotics on *Pneumococcus* these septicemias have a high mortality rate of 53%. Two paradoxical facts appear in the series of Folland *et al.* (1974): (1) leukopenic patients having 1000 white blood cells do not suffer this complication more than those with a normal number of leukocytes; (2) cancer patients with solid tumors, not complicated by lung metastasis, constitute the best target for these septicemias. Some authors consider splenectomy as favoring meningitis and fulminant septicemias caused by pneumococci. Actually, it seems that a splenectomy, which is done for diagnosis and/or therapy, even in malignant lymphomas, does not increase the frequency of superinfections, and rather it is the leukopenia induced by the chemotherapy which plays a major role in the appearance and evolution of bacterial complications, including those caused by pneumococci (Donaldson *et al.*, 1972).

Among the Gram-positive bacilli, *Listeria monocytogenes* deserves the most attention. In addition to its incidence in pregnancy and in the neonatal period, listeriosis readily appears in compromised patients: alcoholics, diabetics, cancerous and immunosuppressed subjects. Listeriosis develops mainly in lymphomas, and particularly in Hodgkin's disease, an illness well characterized by disorders of the cell-mediated immune response (Table XX). In cancer patients it mainly causes septicopyohemias or typhoidlike septicemias and meningitis. In a series of 18 listerioses isolated in malignancies, Louria *et al.* (1967) observed

16 septicemias (9 were complicated by meningitis) and 2 cases of meningitis, but these last two were evidently consequences of a bacteremia. Six of these patients died of these infectious complications.

In some well-documented observations, other Gram-positive bacilli, which are not usually pathogenic, have been considered as being responsible for septicemia in cancer patients. A relapsing septicemia was caused by *Corynebacterium equi* after a lung abscess in a patient suffering a lymphosarcoma (March and Graevenitz, 1973). More recently three bacteremias with previously undescribed species of *Cornyebacterium* have been reported in patients with relapsing leukemia (Hande *et al.*, 1976). Beside a gas gangrene-like infection caused by *Bacillus cereus* in a lymphoma patient (Gröschel *et al.*, 1976), five bacteremias (four with *Bacillus subtilis* and one with *Bacillus cereus*) have been described in patients with acute leukemia: pneumonitis was uniformly present in this group and sputum cultures were positive in all five cases (Sathmary, 1958; Ihde and Armstrong, 1973; Pennington *et al.*, 1976).

## Septicemias Caused by Obligate Anaerobes

These infections are underestimated if the laboratory does not have the appropriate means to detect these organisms, as their isolation and identification are often difficult. When the leukocytic pool is normal there is generally a marked granulocytosis.

Among the spore forming anaerobic microorganisms an infection caused by *Clostridium*, which develops without an obvious portal of entry (such as a wound or a septic abortion), favors the existence of an underlying neoplasm, whether or not the diagnosis of cancer has been established (Alpern and Dowell, 1969). *Clostridium septicum* and *Clostridium perfringens* are most often responsible for septicemias. This complication develops in advanced cancers, particularly those of the digestive tract (Table XXV). The portal of entry is mainly the intestinal tract: effectively, out of 27 cases of infection caused by *Clostridium septicum* a skin lesion was the portal of entry only two times (Alpern and Dowell, 1969.) In these patients the frequency of abdominal pains, nausea, and vomiting, partial or complete intestinal obstruction, even digestive hemorrhages during septicemia, point toward the entry of organisms in the blood stream via intestinal lesions. Three cases of massive hemolysis have been noted in a series of 15 septicemias caused mainly by *Clostridium perfringens* (Wayne and Armstrong, 1972), but only one out of 23 in a series of septicemias was due to *Clostridium septicum* (Alpern and Dowell, 1969). Localized gas crepitus or gas gangrene are seldom seen: out of 23 septicemias caused by *Clostridium septicum*

TABLE XXV.    Distribution of Infections due to Anaerobic Agents According to the Type of Cancer

| Cancers | Clostridium | | Bacteroides | | | |
|---|---|---|---|---|---|---|
| | Central Laboratory, Atlanta (Alpern and Dowell, 1969) | Memorial Hospital, New York (Wynne and Armstrong, 1972) | M.D. Anderson Hospital, Houston (Sinkovics and Smith, 1970) | Memorial Hospital, New York (Kagnoff et al., 1972) | General Hospital, Portsmouth (Okubadejo et al., 1973) | General Hospital, Wycombe (Leigh, 1974) |
| Leukemia | 15 | 3 | 2 | 4 | 0 | 0 |
| Malignant lymphoma | 1 | 3 | 6 | 6 | 0 | 0 |
| Gastrointestinal cancers | 6 | 1 | 7 | 9 | 9 | 12 |
| Other cancers | 2 | 7 | 10 | 32 | 2 | 3 |
| Total | 24 | 14 | 25 | 51 | 11 | 15 |

complicating cancers, there were only two gas gangrene cases (one in a diabetic patient with carcinoma of the caecum, the other in a myelocytic leukemia) which constituted the portals of entry of the systemic infection. Among the 23 septicemias caused by *Clostridium septicum*, 11 were fatal; 9 of them had not received any antibiotics. When the evolution is fatal, it is generally rapid, even fulminating.

In the group of nonsporulated anaerobic microorganisms which constitute the endogenous flora of Veillon, *Bacteroides* most often causes infections and it appears more often to be selected by antibiotics that are used against *Enterobacteriaceae* and the multiresistant *Pseudomonas*. *Bacteroides* are responsible for 2% of the septicemias in neoplastic disease (Sinkovics and Smith, 1970). The main portals of entry are the oropharyngeal area, the gastrointestinal tract, and the female genital tract. These septicemias develop chiefly during solid tumors and particularly in digestive cancers (Table XXV). Recent abdominal or urogenital surgery preceded their development in 58% of the patients of Kagnoff *et al.* (1972). They are complicated by pleuropulmonary localizations: 8 out of 25 cases with 7 fatal evolutions (Sinkovics and Smith, 1970). They were responsible for death in 31% of the cases in the series of Kagnoff *et al.* (1972) and in 72% of the cases in the series of Sinkovics and Smith (1970). The diagnosis of *Bacteroides* infection is not always made during the lifetime of the patient, as these bacteria grow slowly. Finally, we shall mention that besides these anaerobic microorganisms, others such as *Fusobacterium necrophorum* have been recognized as being responsible for septicemias in cancers, especially in digestive tumors (Leng-Levy *et al.*, 1961).

## MYCOBACTERIAL INFECTIONS

### Tuberculosis

Tuberculosis is in definite regression in all countries where the social and economical level is high and it is evident that its incidence in cancer patients is presently low, since the studies concerning this relationship have been done in industrialized countries.

Kaplan *et al.* (1974) reported a large series concerning 201 cancer patients: 77 cases of tuberculosis were diagnosed at the same time the cancer was discovered, 103 when the patients were undergoing anticancer therapy, and 21 developed at a later date.

The common lung cancer and tuberculosis combination was found 44 times. The incidence of this complication is highest in lung cancer, malignant lymphomas, and especially in Hodgkin's disease (Table XXVI).

TABLE XXVI.    Association of Tuberculosis and Cancer[a]

| Cancers | Tuberculosis | | | | | |
| --- | --- | --- | --- | --- | --- | --- |
| | Diagnosis at the Same Time as the Cancer | | | Diagnosis During the Treatment of Cancer | | |
| | Pulmonary Localization | Extrapulmonary Localization | Disseminated Infection | Pulmonary Localization | Extrapulmonary Localization | Disseminated Infection |
| Lung cancers | 24 | 6 | 1 | 12 | 0 | 2 |
| Head and neck cancers | 16 | 3 | 1 | 14 | 0 | 2 |
| Breast cancers | 2 | 5 | 0 | 11 | 1 | 5 |
| Other solid tumors | 11 | 1 | 1 | 17 | 2 | 4 |
| Hodgkin's diseases | 0 | 0 | 1 | 7 | 1 | 6 |
| Other blood malignancy | 5 | 0 | 0 | 9 | 0 | 10 |
| Total | 58 | 15 | 4 | 70 | 4 | 29 |

[a] From Kaplan et al. (1974), 1950–1971, Memorial Hospital, New York, New York.

In lung cancer, the neoplastic lesions may be responsible either for activating a latent preexisting tuberculosis or for the local appearance of an exogenous infection. The importance of tuberculosis lesions during Hodgkin's disease is explained by the impairment of cell-mediated immune response.

Tuberculosis is especially discovered at the same time as the neoplasm in lung cancers and cancers of the head and neck, and, on the other hand, shows up mainly when radiotherapy and chemotherapy have been undertaken in lymphomas and breast cancers.

The main mycobacterial infection is pulmonary tuberculosis. Lymphadenitis and other isolated bacillary localizations, as well as disseminated tuberculosis, are rare.

If the global mortality of tuberculosis is 17%, it is 48% in lymphomas. Nine tuberculosis pneumonias were all fatal and 33 multifocal tuberculoses were fatal in 91% of the cases. Severe pulmonary or disseminated tuberculosis is observed especially during lymphomas and breast cancer under chemotherapy.

## Complications Caused by BCG

Calmette and Guerin attested that bovine tuberculosis bacillus is presently widely used in cancer patients, not as a vaccination against tuberculosis, but rather repeatedly used as an immunologic test or as immunologic stimulation which may be performed on normal skin at a distance from the tumor, or in cutaneous tumor nodules (Sparks et al., 1973); the latter certainly being more hazardous and having a doubtful efficacy. In any case, there is the possibility of transitory bacteremias and the risk of multiple visceral infectious lesions owing to BCG in immunosuppressed subjects and even the possibility of immediate generalized fatal hypersensitivity reactions (Aungst et al., 1975).

The reaction to BCG may involve the scarified cutaneous zone, causing a necrosis, which in our experience has been observed only two times in about 10,000 tests, and easily heals after local application of streptomycin. When BCG is administered in larger doses to provoke an immunologic stimulation on extended scarifications or by intradermal injections, a satellite lymphadenitis of the injected territory is usually seen. Sometimes it develops and fistulizes, giving pus which is full of acid-fast bacilli. It is a complication that we have observed two times in 70 patients, each one being submitted to about 100 large scarifications. Moreover, in these two cases in order to bring about retrocession and healing it was enough to stop the applications in the corresponding areas (Hoerni et al., 1976). These scarifications are frequently accompanied by a febrile reaction that might be linked to a bacteremia which has actually been affirmed and are favored by immunosuppression; generalized complications such as pulmonary miliary or hepatic granulomatosis are rare (Sparks *et al.*, 1973). Finally, in immunocompetent patients, delayed hypersensitivity reactions, with important local lesions, fever, even erythema nodosum, have seldom been reported (Aungst *et al.*, 1975).

## Atypical Mycobacteriosis

These cause pulmonary and lymph-node lesions, or sometimes multiple and disseminated lesions identical to those of tuberculosis and for the moment, they are still rare. Tuberculin allergy is generally absent. These mycobacteria, different from Hansen's bacillus and from human or bovine tuberculosis bacilli, are mainly found in nature and become pathogenic by accident. They are identified by their rapid growth on Löwenstein–Jensen medium, by their colonial morphology, and by their biochemical characteristics.

From 1968 to 1973, Feld *et al.* (1976) found mycobacteriosis in 59 patients with malignant disease; among them 30 patients (51%) had mycobacteriosis caused by atypical mycobacteria. The most frequent organisms were *Mycobacterium kansasii* and *Mycobacterium fortuitum.* The most frequent cancers associated with these mycobacteria were testicular carcinoma, head and neck squamous cell carcinoma, lymphoma, and lung carcinoma. The only predisposing factor was cancer chemotherapy.

Some other well-documented observations of atypical mycobacteriosis have been reported. Infiltrated and excavated lesions in both lungs caused by *Mycobacterium kansasii* have been observed in a patient with Hodgkin's disease in remission but with an impairment of immunologic functions; they healed completely with appropriate antibiotic treatment. The same mycobacteriosis caused by *Mycobacterium kansasii*, disseminated and of fatal evolution, with, in particular pleuropulmonary, splenic, lymph-node and bone-marrow localizations, has been reported during a chronic myeloid leukemia (Grillo-Lopez *et al.*, 1971). *Mycobacterium kansasii* was also isolated from the spleen of a patient with hairy-cell leukemia, who had caseating necrosis of the spleen and liver and probably had involvement of the lung (Manes and Blair, 1976).

Because of the present regression of tuberculosis, these atypical mycobacterial infections should be more readily considered (despite their rarity) together with a clinical picture of tuberculosis. They are resistant to isoniaizde but are sensitive to rifampicin, ethambutol, and cycloserine.

This chapter has underlined the main characteristics of bacterial infections during cancer: their frequency, the predominance of Gram-negative bacilli (particularly *Pseudomonas*), and the importance and the gravity of these frequently lethal complications.

It is important to emphasize that malignant blood diseases, which are in an advanced stage, and generalized solid tumors are particularly susceptible to these superinfections. The clinical aspect of these bacterial infections is rather uniform. It is characterized by fever and signs of localization that are not always clinically evident. As we have seen in Chapter 4 it is necessary to always recall the possibility of these infections and to give early therapy to patients who may rapidly die from infectious shock or severe pneumonia. Antibiotic treatment, even when it is appropriate, is not always successful. Too often the compromised status of these patients, especially a severe granulocytopenia, is responsible for a poor prognosis.

# CHAPTER 6

# Viral Infections

The relationships between cancer and viruses are complex and are difficult for several reasons. Because of the ubiquity of viruses their detection, by direct means or indirectly by serodiagnosis, is often subject to various interpretations. In addition, the reaction of a given virus with a cell, a tissue, or an organism varies depending on several factors as shown in the following example. The Epstein–Barr virus is certainly responsible for benign cellular proliferation that corresponds to infectious mononucleosis, an illness which varies from an inapparent infection to some particularly severe forms; the same agent seems to play the role of a co-factor at the onset of cancers such as Burkitt's lymphoma or nasopharyngeal carcinoma. Finally, one may find it as a latent and opportunistic superinfecting agent in immunosuppressed patients.

Schematically, the relationships between viruses and cancers may be seen from two different points of view, although some are difficult to classify.

## Viruses as the Cause of Cancers

There is no definite proof that a virus causes cancer in man. However, certain observations seem to imply that a virus may play a role, at least as a co-factor, in the genesis of some tumors.

Thus, the Epstein–Barr virus was accused, even before it was identified, as the etiologic agent of Burkitt's lymphoma, then later of nasopharyngeal carcinoma observed especially in the south of China. Its constant isolation in neoplastic cells of these cancers has not yet demonstrated either if, or how, this virus intervenes (Burkitt and Wright, 1970; Liabeuf and Kourilsky, 1975; De-Thé et al., 1975).

More recently herpes simplex virus type-2 has been implicated in the genesis of carcinoma of the cervix uteri (Symposium 1973; Melnick and Rawls, 1974) and its homolog type-1 for lip and mouth cancers.

Finally, we shall cite the problems raised by the observation of Hb antigen (Australia) in malignant hepatomas, which give some support to the theory that chronic infection by hepatitis B virus could play a role, at least in certain cases and along with other factors, in the origin of hepatic carcinomas (Bourgeaux et al., 1973; Maupas et al., 1975).

These data do not deal directly with our topic. They are only mentioned in the context of where the virus may be found once the cancer has developed. The virus may be found in the neoplastic cells or in their environment, either directly under a complete form, or indirectly (by way of antibodies, from a culture result or by nucleic acid hybridization). Such findings may thus not be due to a superinfection of the cancer or of the cancer patient, but may only correspond to the persistence of an infectious state prior to the tumor. On the contrary, electron microscopic observation of viral particles in cancer cells, which was very popular 10 years ago, does not positively signify that the observed virus has any carcinogenic responsibility (see Chapter 1).

## Superinfection in Cancer Patients

A viral infection in a cancer patient may be inapparent and discovered only by routine examination, or it may be responsible for apparent clinical manifestations. We shall discuss the first possibility before analyzing different viroses in detail.

The traces of an inapparent virosis are generally sought for by systematic serodiagnosis.

Because of its relations with Burkitt's lymphoma, the Epstein–Barr virus has been sought for in other lymphomas. Alongside of negative studies (Goldman and Aisenberg, 1970; Hirshaut et al., 1974), an increase, in relation to a control population, of the median titer of antibodies against this virus has been found in patients with malignant lymphoma and especially in Hodgkin's disease (particularly in the lymphoid depletion form) (Johansson et al., 1970; Levine et al., 1971). At the same time, the antibody titers against herpes-virus hominis types 1 and 2, cytomegalovirus, and varicella virus were normal, while other authors observed an increase of antibodies against herpes-virus type-2 in Hodgkin's disease of a mixed cellularity type (Catalano and Goldman, 1972). The responsibility of an immunologic factor was suspected because of the affinity for Hodgkin's patients, who present an immune deficiency that is particularly marked in case of lymphoid depletion. This has been supported by comparable observation during sarcoidosis, which is characterized by the same type of immune deficiency (Hirshaut et al., 1970). The fact that this para-Hodgkin's or parasarcoidosis immune deficiency involves cell-mediated immunity and respects humoral immunity (consequently, the researched antibodies) should not be forgotten. Hesse et al. (1973) did not observe any variation in the diverse types of antibodies against the Epstein–Barr virus in the evolution of Hodgkin's disease or in chronic lymphoid leukemia, while Langenhuysen *et al.* (1974) observed an increase in various antiviral antibodies with the aggravation of Hodgkin's disease. They attributed this to a humoral hyperactivity, secondarily to the impaired cell-mediated immune response. It is striking to observe that high antibody titers are seen in chronic lymphoid leukemia, but not in chronic myeloid leukemia (Levine *et al.*, 1971).

Research of Hb antigen prevalence has given similar results (Sutnick *et al.*, 1970). The presence of this antigen is more frequent in Hodgkin's patients or patients with acute leukemia or chronic lymphoid leukemia, and less in patients with chronic myeloid leukemia. It is linked to prior transfusions and characterized by its persistence. This chronic and latent infection is also related to the immune deficiency of the patients, which is paraneoplastic and eventually is maintained or aggravated by maintenance therapy. However, it is not always completely inapparent, for systematic examinations link it to an increase of serum glutamopyruvic transaminases, a disturbance of the bromsulfalein test, and histologic lesions compatible with a persistent chronic hepatitis (Grange *et al.*, 1975). Some virus-like particles have been observed in hepatic cells of seropositive patients (Nowoslawski *et al.*, 1970). The recent publication of Galbraith *et al.* (1975) gives further evidence that particular attention should be given to systematic research of that latent viral infection. These authors observed three fatal cases of hepatitis when chemotherapy was discontinued: they think that the discontinuation of the therapy permits a recovery of immunologic reactions against the virus and that this facilitates the formation of antigen–antibody complexes which cause a massive destruction of hepatic cells. If these theories are confirmed, they would imply that particular precautions need to be taken when therapy is discontinued in patients carrying this antigen. These leukemia patients, who harbor Hb antigen, may be a source of infection and are sometimes responsible for other cases in their contacts (Steinberg *et al.*, 1975). Such data show that the presence of Hb antigen is not only a latent infection but may be the source of mild or more severe disease.

Viral hepatitis, often latent, sometimes overt, leads us into a discussion on viral diseases, dominated by herpes virus infections.

## HERPES ZOSTER AND VARICELLA

### Etiology

The common and easily identifiable infections have a prominent place in publications, but this may be misleading, for most other viroses are more difficult to recognize. The principal series reported these past few years are indicated in Table V. Most authors agree that herpes zoster is due to a varicella virus that has remained dormant in the spinal ganglions. Moreover, the history of a previous infection by varicella is found in the majority of patients with herpes zoster; but Schimpff *et al.* (1972), during an epidemic of varicella and herpes zoster, reported observations compatible with the direct propagation of varicella-zoster virus from one patient to another resulting in clinical herpes zoster.

The mechanisms which favor the development of such infections have been discussed in Chapter 3. We shall recall the important role of paraneoplastic immune deficiency which is affirmed by comparing Hodgkin's disease and non-Hodgkin's lymphomas (Chauvergne *et al.*, 1969; Hoerni *et al.*, 1972), or the histologic subtypes of Hodgkin's disease (Monfardini *et al.*, 1973). The infection sometimes precedes the diagnosis of cancer by a few months, and its development in a young adult can raise suspicion of Hodgkin's disease. This deficiency could also explain relapsing herpes zoster, which ranges from several months to intervals of years as we have observed in several patients. The role of radiotherapy is widely appreciated, as well as that of heavy chemotherapy or splenectomy (Goffinet *et al.*, 1972; Monfardini *et al.*, 1973). Since the intensity of the treatment is generally proportional to the extension of the illness, it seems difficult to define precisely the responsibilities. However, in a small series of 133 patients with Hodgkin's disease, clinical stage I or II, observed between 1966 and 1974, the first group of patients had been treated only by radiotherapy, whereas the following group had been treated by radiotherapy along with one or several courses of chemotherapy (Durand *et al.*, 1976). No increase in the frequency of herpes zoster was observed for patients with chemotherapy (Table XXVII). One may, however, define a group of high-risk patients. Thus, patients with stages III and IV Hodgkin's disease, with an anergy to dinitrochlorobenzene (DNCB), and who have re-

TABLE XXVII. Frequency of Herpes Zoster in Clinical Stage I and II Hodgkin's Disease According to the Treatment[a]

| Treatment | Number of Patients | Number of Infections |
|---|---|---|
| Radiotherapy only | 42 | 7 |
| Radiotherapy + chemotherapy (1 course) | 23 | 6 |
| Radiotherapy + chemotherapy (2 courses or more) | 68 | 9 |
| Total | 133 | 22 |

[a] 1965–1974, Cancer Center, Bordeaux, France.

cently received total lymph-node irradiation, have 62 chances out of 100 to develop zoster (Schimpff et al., 1972). In our experience concerning hematologic neoplasms, herpes virus infection occurs mainly in the complete remission stage of Hodgkin's disease, and in the evolutive stage (first stage or relapse) for other malignancies (Table XXVIII). Since adjuvant chemotherapy for localized breast cancer has been used, it seems that there are many herpes zoster cases in these patients, while this virosis was very rare in patients with the same cancer when they were treated only by surgery with or without radiotherapy.

## Herpes Zoster

The clinical aspect of herpes zoster does not differ in cancer patients from the usual aspect (Juel-Jensen and MacCallum, 1972). Thoracic regions are involved in one out of two patients (Goffinet et al., 1972), but any other region is susceptible (Fig. 9). In our experience ophthalmic localization appears less frequently (3%) in cancer patients than in the general population. Localizations have been reported in the Hunt's area (Shanbrom et al., 1960). Moreover, in these patients herpes zoster complications readily set in, either locally or systematically. Locally these lesions may become infected by lack of local hygiene, the same as in non–cancer patients. More particular is the confluence (Fig. 10) which may lead to a necrosis of large cutaneous areas in the corresponding dermatome. The hemorrhagic character of the vesicles depends on local or general conditions, such as thrombocytopenia or various hemostatic disorders. Generalization is more severe; estimated at 4% in the general population (Bodey, 1975) and it is clearly more frequent (from 30 to 40%) in cancer patients (Sokal and Firat, 1965; Schimpff et al., 1972). The clinical aspect generally consists of a high fever with a severe alteration of the general status which may cause death. Other complications of herpes zoster, such as neurologic ones, have neither a particular frequency nor character in cancer patients; we have observed, with exception, important pain sequela. While in a healthy child the infection, which represents 5% of all herpes zoster, has almost always a benign course (Rogers and Tindall, 1972), in children with cancer its evolution is most often severe (Muller, 1967) and can be complicated, especially by pneumonia, meningoencephalitis, thrombocytopenia, iritis, or keratitis (Feldman et al., 1977). Complicated herpes zoster may, in itself, have a certain gravity, but its development is above all a sign of poor prognosis in the evolution of malignant blood diseases (Sokal, 1966; Hoerni et al., 1972). On the contrary, herpes zoster, which develops in the 6 months following diagnosis and initial treatment, does not have any influence on the prognosis (see Chapter 11).

TABLE XXVIII.  Evolutive Stage of Blood Malignancy at the Moment
of Herpes Virus Infection[a]

| Hematologic Neoplasm | Perceptible Phase | | Complete Remission | Total |
|---|---|---|---|---|
| | Stages I and II | Stages III and IV | | |
| Hodgkin's disease | 7 | 10 | 40 | 57 |
| Non-Hodgkin's lymphoma | 9 | 16 | 7 | 32 |
| Leukemia | 0 | 7 | 2 | 9 |
| Total | 16 | 33 | 49 | 98 |

From Durand *et al.* (1976), 1960–1974; Cancer Center, Bordeaux, France.

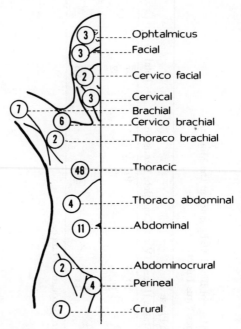

**Fig. 9.**   Localizations of 100 herpes zoster occurring in patients with malignant lymphoma.

## Varicella

As in the general population, varicella particularly affects children and thus it is most often associated with leukemias, which represent one-fourth of children's neoplasms, and because of its contagiousness, is feared in hematologic pediatric services. Its constant benignity in normal children is not found in leukemic patients, who may succumb to the illness: out of 34 infections, 18 had a benign evolution, but 11 were severe and 5 fatal (Schaison *et al.*, 1971). Severe forms are characterized by large size, numerous, and hemorrhagic vesicles covering the entire body, particularly the palms and the soles, and sometimes the cornea and larynx (which usually remain free) and they are accompanied by marked systemic symptoms. Fatal forms depend on a generalization of the virus in the host with, in particular, a neurologic syndrome and diffuse hemorrhagic signs, linked to a thrombocytopenia and/or disseminated intravascular coagulation. Rare pulmonary varicella may simulate metastatic deposits (Domart *et al.*, 1964; Adenis *et al.*, 1975). This virus is considered as responsible for some allergic granulomatosis (Rosenblum and Hadfield, 1972). Pro-

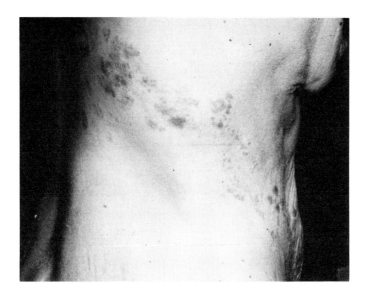

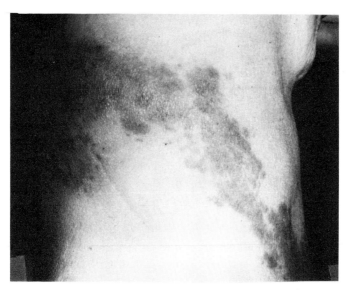

**Fig. 10.** Thoracoabdominal herpes zoster evolving towards confluence in a 45-year-old woman with advanced Hodgkin's disease.

longed corticosteroids seem to accentuate the viremia and favor the development of a severe infection; the stage of the leukemia also conditions the severity of the infection (Bodey *et al.*, 1964). However, there is no strict correlation between malignant blood disease or its treatment and the severity of the virosis. In this uncertainty, the importance attached to prophylactic treatment (which will be discussed in Chapter 9) is readily comprehensible. In the absence of a regularly efficacious curative treatment the only action generally recommended is to continue corticosteroids when the infection breaks out during such treatment (Schaison *et al.*, 1971), although this suggestion is not supported by solid evidence.

## Treatment

The curative treatment of herpes zoster and varicella can be considered simultaneously. The administration of nonspecific gamma globulins, formerly proposed, is very debatable, and usually has been abandoned. On the contrary, specific immunoglobulins are very useful (Gaiffe *et al.*, 1976). We shall only mention common treatments, such as emetine, or more recent ones, such as amantadine (Galbraith, 1973), whose efficacy is difficult to affirm. Cytarabine (or cytosine-arabinoside or cara-C), which was at first and is still employed as an antileukemic agent and whose toxicity is not negligible (Karchmer and Hirsch, 1973), acts on the virus by inhibiting DNA synthesis, but its usefulness in the treatment of these infections has not been demonstrated (Davis *et al.*, 1973). Some reports are in favor of its efficacy (McKelvey and Kwaan, 1969), especially for ophthalmic herpes zoster (Pierce and Jenkins, 1973), but a controlled study concerning generalized herpes zoster in Hodgkin's patients shows that the evolution of the cutaneous lesions is prolonged in comparison to patients receiving a placebo. This could be explained by an immunosuppressive effect (Stevens *et al.*, 1973); however, this failure may be linked to the fact that cytarabine is administered too late after the onset of the infection, at the moment of generalization. In all cases local care should reduce the risks of superinfection. Continuous application of idoxuridine on skin lesions reduces pain and significantly accelerates healing in comparison with intermittent application (Juel-Jensen *et al.*, 1970).

More recently adenine-arabinoside (ara-A) has been used because it has a therapeutic index which is better than that of ara-C. Preliminary results have been reported from a controlled and cooperative study including 87 patients, the majority of them suffering a malignant lymphoma: the decrease of pain and the healing of skin lesions are more rapid in treated patients than in untreated ones; the late effects are difficult to appreciate. The therapeutic improvement seems better than with ara-C, mainly because of a lesser toxicity (Ch'ien *et al.*, 1976).

## OTHER INFECTIONS CAUSED BY HERPES VIRUS

Infections caused by type-1 *Herpes virus hominis*, in the respiratory and digestive tracts, or by type-2 in the genital regions, are characterized by clusters of vesicles, inflamed and persistent, mainly involving the lips, nose, mouth, or genital mucous membrane (Fig. 11). But, herpetic infection may spread to the mucous membranes of the respiratory and digestive tracts and frequently can cause esophagitis (Weiden and Schuffler, 1974) or tracheobronchitis. They readily have a chronic evolution, but generalization is rare (Lynfield *et al.*, 1969). The severest complication is an exudative pneumonia (Rosen and Hajdu, 1971). A few cases of herpes simplex encephalitis have been observed in patients with carcinoma of the uterus (Dayan *et al.*, 1967) or with Hodgkin's disease (Heineman and Breen, 1975).

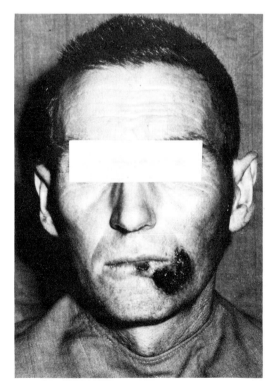

**Fig. 11.** Labial herpes in a 47-year-old patient suffering from Hodgkin's disease with massive liver involvement.

Herpetic infection seems to be often overlooked, even ignored, since systematic viral examination isolates the virus in 16% of patients with malignant blood diseases and in 58% of those who present a buccal ulceration (Aston et al., 1972). The diagnostic proof of such an infection is effectively difficult to affirm, especially if the clinical aspect does not raise suspicion. Isolation of the virus on a culture of HeLa cells is essential; 5% of patients without erosive lesion, but who carry the virus, can also be found with this method; this percentage is close to that found in the general population. Biopsy of mucous lesions may sometimes show giant multinucleated cells characteristic of the infection (Weiden and Schuffler, 1974). Antemortem diagnosis of herpetic esophagitis may be made by brush cytology when the esophagoscopy is performed (Lightdale et al., 1977).

The lesions may respond favorably to irradiation (Aston et al., 1972) or more usually to idoxuridine, particularly useful in herpetic keratitis (it should be applied several times every day), but this drug is poorly tolerated when administered intravenously and its efficacy has not been established by controlled studies (Weinstein and Chang, 1973). This infection is, in itself, sometimes severe, but often corresponds to a poor prognosis of the underlying hematologic malignancy (Hoerni et al., 1972). Some cases of esophagitis resolved when the patient responded to anticancer therapy, regardless of the tumor site (Lightdale et al., 1977).

*Cytomegalovirus* is a common virus; 80% of the adult population possess complement-fixing antibodies. Pathologic manifestations caused by this virus are rare: the clinical picture is variable, characterized mainly by a mononucleosis, typically by its clinical and hematologic features, and often with hepatic and pulmonary disorders (Aubertin et al., 1972; Dao, 1973). In cancer patients the infection can be either latent or discrete: systematic serodiagnosis performed in 27 leukemic patients demonstrated six positive conversions and four important increases in the antibody titer accompanied by an excretion of virus (Caul et al., 1972). The rate of positivity increases with the duration of the observation (Sullivan et al., 1968). Interhuman transmission or transmission by transfusion would be responsible, but isolation of patients is without effect (Cox and Hughes, 1975). Sometimes the virosis is at the origin of serious clinical manifestations that are diagnosed at necropsy by the presence of intranuclear inclusions in the large cells observed in the lungs and other organs. Presently, an effort must be made to identify this virus by serodiagnosis while the patient is alive. The clinical picture is dominated by an almost constant fever, hepatic lesions which are generally subclinical (Bussel et al., 1975), a pneumonia (Cangir et al., 1967), and more rarely by a splenomegaly or cutaneous rash. According to the data of a small series of 16 cytomegalovirus pneumonias, Abdallah *et al.* (1976) emphasize the difficulties of the diagnosis, which was made in 11 living patients only by bronchoaspiration or pulmonary biopsy. They also noted a frequent association between cytomegalovirus and either *Pneumocystis carinii*, fungus, or Koch's bacillus at the origin of the pneumonia. One case of acute colitis in a patient with acute lymphoid leukemia has been reported (Beaugrand *et al.*, 1976). It is often associated with a blood pancytopenia and bone marrow aplasia and rather often with a monoclonal gammapathy (Vodopick *et al.*, 1974). Briefly, the picture is often that of a hematologic malignancy in as far as an eventual lymph-node biopsy may reveal alterations resembling malignant lymphoma. The possibility of this virosis being present should systematically be considered and affirmed by the repetition of complement-fixation tests, or better, either by direct hemagglutination or by isolation of the virus from the leukocytic fraction of the patient's blood (Bussel *et al.*, 1975). It is important to affirm this diagnosis because useless treatments can be avoided, in particular broad spectrum antibiotics. Even if some antiviral chemotherapeutic studies have been reported, the main treatment seems to be the discontinuation of the maintenance chemotherapy (which is generally handicapped by the leukopenia), for the evolution is most often spontaneously favorable (Bussel *et al.*, 1975).

The rare observations of infectious mononucleosis (Massey *et al.*, 1953; Kenis *et al.*, 1959) are disputable, for on the one hand Hodgkin's disease, during which they were observed, is suspected of being accompanied by a mononucleosis, and on the other hand, falsely positive serodiagnoses have been observed in cancer patients, particularly those with lymphoma (Wolf *et al.*, 1970; Sadoff and Goldsmith, 1971).

## OTHER VIRAL INFECTIONS

Measles affects children with cancer above all, but appears much less frequently since young children are routinely vaccinated. Generally, it does not have any particular aspect, but pulmonary and otorhinolaryngeal superinfections are rather frequent and fatal pneumonias have been observed. Some particular cases have been reported: one giant cell pneumonia and two cases of lethal encephalopathy in three children in complete remission during maintenance chemotherapy (Pullan *et al.*, 1976) and two encephalopathies, whose clinical picture was similar to that of sclerosing panencephalitis (Smyth *et al.*, 1976). It has been reported that this virus remains in the throat of leukemic patients several weeks after the illness (Bodey, 1975), and some cases have been terminated fatally (Breitfeld *et al.*, 1973).

The "flu" is probably one of the most frequent viral infections; unfortunately there are few publications concerning it. Recently, Feldman *et al.* (1977) reported 20 cases of influenza diagnosed by serodiagnosis in cancer patients less than 23 years old (14 hematologic malignancies and 6 solid tumors). The clinical picture differed from the usual picture by a longer duration (1–2 weeks) of the symptoms (fever, cough, coryza, myalgy, headache). Complications were observed only in three patients regardless of the form of cancer or the type of treatment. The most important consequence of this common infection is that anticancer treatment is temporarily interrupted in the majority of the cases. Mumps and adenovirosis do not usually have any predilection for children with cancer in comparison with healthy children.

Viral hepatitis does not seem to have either a particular frequency or a particular clinical aspect in cancer patients, except for an infection which is often latent as mentioned previously. Some observations of systemic vaccinia, even fatal, have been reported following an untimely vaccination against variola (see Chapter 9).

Rare progressive multifocal leukoencephalopathy is due to a viral infection of the oligodendroglia which causes demyelination. The responsible virus is morphologically very close to the polyoma-SV 40 subgroup of the papovaviruses: ZuRhein and Chou (1965) first demonstrated viral particles by electron microscopy; then Padgett *et al.* (1971) isolated a JC virus from the brain, which has been confirmed by other researchers (Narayan *et al.*, 1973). The clinical aspect is characterized by a fever of long duration, accompanied by progressive paralysis leading to death in about 12 months. Computed tomography may be an aid in the diagnosis (Carroll *et al.*, 1977). Most encephalopathies have been reported during immunologic deficiencies or hematologic malignancies, especially in Hodgkin's disease and chronic lymphoid leukemia (Weiner *et al.*, 1973). The efficacy of cytarabine in their treatment has not been precisely demonstrated (Conomy *et al.*, 1974). Only a few cases have been reported in which the patients recovered after treatment with cytarabine (Buckman and Wiltshaw, 1976).

In conclusion, viroses such as herpes zoster, varicella, herpes simplex, cytomegalic inclusion disease, and vaccinia can produce severe infections in cancer patients, particularly those with hematologic malignancies, whereas others, such as those caused by rhinoviruses, adenoviruses, and enteroviruses, are observed in cancer patients as well as in healthy subjects, with the same frequency and clinical course (Schaison *et al.*, 1971; Feldman and Cox, 1976). Viral hepatitis, which is frequent but rarely severe, constitutes a transitory virosis. The causes of these variations are unknown, but perhaps these observations may contribute to a better understanding of the defense reactions against viruses.

# CHAPTER 7

# Fungal Infections

These are typical opportunistic infections (Klastersky, 1972). The responsible agents are microorganisms that are usually saprophytic but, at the occasion of an impairment of host defense mechanisms, have become pathogenic. Fungal infections, localized in healthy individuals, tend to disseminate in cancer patients. The diagnosis and treatment of these infections are often difficult, hence their prognosis is often poor.

## GENERAL INFORMATION

### Frequency

Fungal infections occupy an important place in the infectious pathology of cancer patients. For example, in the series of Levine *et al.* (1972), which concerns only hematologic malignancies, focalized or septicemic fungal infections represent 31% of the 462 infections which had developed in 354 necropsied patients. Actually, the exact incidence of fungal infections can only be judged on necropsied series. Infections revealed at necropsies are much more numerous than those diagnosed when the patients are alive; in addition, the frequency of fungal isolation in cancer patients does not necessarily reflect an infection in these subjects, as fungal saprophytism is common.

These views need to be defined in relation to the general incidence of fungal infections. The general population carries fungi relatively frequently, but these microorganisms seldom cause pathological manifestations. Thus, in the study of Toala *et al.* (1970), the isolation of *Candida* represented 0.78% of all microbiologically positive cultures; these fungi came from 151 patients of whom only 56 had clinical manifestations of fungal infection and among these, 25% had cancers. These facts are confirmed in other series (Moulinier *et al.*, 1972) and for other fungi; only 40% of subjects who are carriers of *Coccidioides* have infectious symptoms (Deresinski and Stevens, 1974). Out of 167 isolations of *Torulopsis* there were only 27 infections (Aisner *et al.*, 1976).

All cancers do not seem to have the same propensity to favor the development of fungal infections. Excluding cutaneous and digestive candidiasis, which are readily observed in patients with solid tumors, other fungal infections together with visceral or disseminated candidiasis are twice as frequent during malignant blood diseases and especially in acute leukemias (Krick and Remington, 1976).

Cancer patients are excellent hosts for fungal infection, but they are not the only ones. All studies insist on the frequency of fungal infections in patients previously treated by antibiotics. There does not seem to be any particular antibiotic which favors fungal infection. Corticosteroids favor *Candida* infection, but are not essential for its development (Levine *et al.*, 1972; Bodey, 1975).

The incidence of fungal infection is not the same for all fungi. In a previous study Zimmerman (1955) distinguished (i) the frequent infections caused by *Candida, Aspergillus,* or mucorales (their increasing number appeared to be proportional to the acquisition of new anticancer therapies); (ii) other fungal infections, such as histoplasmosis or cryptococcosis, whose frequency increased only in patients with leukemia or lymphoma; (iii) a third group, constituted by blastomycosis, sporotrichosis, chromoblastosis, coccidioidomycosis, maduromycosis, which cause only sporadic infections. Bodey (1975) proposes two categories of fungal infection: (1) the first group includes fungal infections caused by saprophytes, such as *Candida, Aspergillus, Phycomycetes, Torulopsis,* and *Geotrichum*; they are rarely responsible for infections in normal individuals but may become pathogenic in severely immunodepressed patients; (2) The second group includes infections caused by *Cryptococcus, Histoplasma,* and *Coccidioides.* These are already a source of infection in the general population and they readily provoke generalized infections in cancer patients, which probably correspond to the reactivation of latent infections, malignant lymphomas being particularly susceptible.

Epidemiology varies according to the region; for example, in comparison with the United States, France has at least three groups of fungal infections which may be individualized: candidiasis is by far the most numerous; aspergillosis and cryptococcosis are rarer than the aforementioned, but are more frequent than in the past; finally, all other fungal infections are only sporadic, probably because of their rarity in Europe.

## Clinical Aspects and Diagnosis

Some common characteristics of various fungal infections should be noted.

In cancer patients, fungal infection may present three different aspects: (1) a superficial disease by direct inoculation is typically represented by cutaneous and mucous membrane candidiasis, but also by candidiasis of the urinary or pulmonary tract; (2) disseminated infection causes a septicemia; (3) visceral invasion involves pulmonary, cerebral, renal, or other parenchyma via the blood stream. These latter localizations, regardless of the fungal agent, create nonspecific syndromes, and are analogous to those of other infections. Hence it is difficult to differentiate between them. This is particularly true for pulmonary localizations, but may also be found in other foci which may, in addition, be clinically latent.

These clinical diagnostic difficulties are linked to those of identifying the fungi. It is easy to prove digestive candidiasis by an appropriate specimen, to identify a septicemia caused by *Candida* by blood cultures, to isolate *Cryptococcus* from a spinal fluid; however, it is much more difficult to confirm pulmonary aspergillosis, histoplasmosis, or mucosmycosis. Bone marrow cultures may sometimes be useful (Hughes, 1971). The presence of fungus in sputum or bronchial specimen is not sufficient to affirm a fungal infection (Levine *et al.*, 1971). In some cases, specific antibodies are found in the patient's serum, but their interpretation is not always clear (Bodey, 1975). In other circumstances only the isolation of the fungus in histologic examinations confirms the diagnosis. It is exceptional to demonstrate *Cryptococccs* at the direct examination of a bone marrow biopsy (O'Carroll *et al.*, 1976). Hence, the difference which has been emphasized between the number of clinically diagnosed fungal infections and the number of infections revealed only at necropsy is explained.

## Treatment

Superficial fungal infections are often sensitive only to topical application of antiseptics or antibiotics. On the contrary, many deep or disseminated visceral mycoses poorly respond to general treatment. There are some active products, but their number is limited; amphotericin B, nystatin, flucytosine, and clotrimazole. The possibilities of application are restrained owing to the reduced diffusibility of nystatin and amphotericin, a serious toxicity for amphotericin, a relatively narrow spectrum of action for flucytosine (Bennett, 1974). Clotrimazole seems to be an interesting drug since its efficacy is better *in vitro* than that of amphotericin B and flucytosine for *Coccidioides, Candida,* and *Cryptococcus* (Hoeprich and Huston, 1975). Moreover, there is a synergistic activity between amphotericin B and flucytosine for *Candida* (Montgomerie *et al.*, 1975), while for other fungi these two drugs may have an independent or antagonist activity (Shadony *et al.*, 1975). Finally, the fungal lesion in itself is often composed of poorly vascularized tissue in infarcted zones, which prevents the penetration of antibiotics into the center of the infectious foci. In a few cases surgical excision has improved these insufficiencies, but the indications are rare.

## CANDIDIASIS

### Etiology

*Candida albicans* is responsible in 75% of the cases of candidiasis and *Candida tropicalis* in 20% (Louria *et al.*, 1962). Other species which have more rarely been observed are *Candida krusei, C. parakrusei*, and *C. guilliermondi*, etc.

Between 30 and 70% of the population carries *Candida.* From 35% in healthy individuals, the frequency of digestive carriers rapidly increases in hospitalized patients, being higher when the hospitalization is longer and the patient receives antibiotic therapy (Aubertin and Leng, 1973). The portal of entry of these infections is generally digestive, but may also be urinary or venous (by catheters).

Candidiasis is observed in all forms of cancers, but has a preference for acute leukemias (Bodey, 1966; Eras *et al.*, 1972). It may occur at any time during the evolution of the cancer; it usually appears late in non-ulcerated visceral cancers in the generalized state with cachexia and early in ulcerated cancers it coexists with intense granulopenia in leukemias. It is almost always secondary to antibiotic therapy (Levine *et al.*, 1972). It is also favored by a functional deficiency of granulocytes, characteristic of Hodgkin's disease, leukemias, and of patients treated by chemotherapy for advanced cancer. The granulocytic deficit is mainly one of the phagocytic activity and the possibilities of fungal lysis; it can be linked to an endocellular deficiency in lysozyme and myeloperoxydase (Lehrer and Cline, 1971).

### Clinical Aspects

The most frequent localizations are superficial. In the mouth, candidiasis provokes stomatitis, glossitis, pharyngitis, easily recognized owing to the pulpy coating which covers a red mucous membrane. Anal localization produces an erythematous area, sometimes runny, which is limited by an epidermal detachment. These lesions can cause important discomfort for the patient.

Candidiasis can also affect the digestive tract—the stomach as well as the intestinal tract. Symptoms may be evident, or, on the contrary, completely absent. Fungal infection is detected only at necropsy in 2% of solid tumors, 10% of lymphomas, and 15% of acute leukemias (Eras *et al.*, 1972). Esophagitis may be manifested by thoracic pains and dysphagia. Radiologic investigation sometimes shows an irregular aspect of the mucous membrane. Esophagoscopy shows pseudomembranous or ulcerated lesions with more or less distinct parietal infiltration. The nutritional consequence is important, complications such as hemorrhages and perforations can be produced (Moulinier et al., 1972). Colon involvement is more discrete, even though it may provoke abdominal pains, diarrhea, and sometimes hemorrhages.

Urinary and pulmonary infections are derived from either a direct inoculation or via the blood stream and then are included in the context of septicemic dissemination. Urinary candidiasis is often asymyptomatic and only identified by examination of urine; however, it is sometimes responsible for cystitis or pyelonephritis.

Respiratory fungal infection often follows bacterial infection (Bodey, 1975). It may assume the aspect of a bronchitis (Lacoste and Mandoul, 1971), or a pneumonia, but the clinical and radiologic symptomatology is not specific. The clinical picture may simulate a localization of a cancer or a viral or parasitic infection. The diagnosis is often suspected owing to the ineffectiveness of antibiotic treatment.

Septicemias are secondary to intravenous catheters or to superficial localization. Highly febrile, they are not clinically specific, but the failure to respond to antibiotic therapy should arouse suspicion of fungal infection, which is easily confirmed by blood cultures. They sometimes disappear with the simple removal of the catheter, which was the initial cause of the infection.

Hematologic dissemination leads to multiple metastasis. All series which mention necropsies indicate the frequency of clinically unsuspected visceral invasions. The small intestine, colon, kidney, bladder, prostrate, thyroid, liver, spleen, heart, and gall bladder may be involved (Mirsky and Cuttner, 1972). Multiple muscle localizations have been observed in a patient with acute lymphoid leukemia (Diggs et al., 1976). A splenic candidiasis has been accompanied by hypersplenism (Bodey et al., 1969). In many cases fungal cultures taken while the patient was alive were negative: only 25% of patients with disseminated candidiasis have positive blood cultures (Bodey, 1966).

Meningitis or meningoencephalitis caused by Candida gives a clear cerebrospinal fluid with a varied cell count, an increased protein concentration, and decreased sugar concentration, but this also is not specific, and only direct examination or culture can affirm the diagnosis.

## Diagnosis

The diagnosis of visceral candidiasis is clinically difficult. Blood cultures are rarely positive. Because of the ubiquity of these fungi their isolation in sputum, on skin, in saliva, or urine does not signify that they are responsible for an infection. However, Bodey (1966) estimates that the presence of *Candida* simultaneously in the urine, saliva, and stools of a febrile and neutropenic patient has a 60% chance to correspond to an infection.

The demonstration of visceral candidiasis, unifocal or disseminated, is based on anticandida antibodies (Rosner *et al.*, 1971) or on histologic examination of a biopsy (Fig. 12). However, serology is not always reliable as anticandida precipitins or agglutinins may be lacking in patients with superficial candidiasis (Wegmann *et al.*, 1971) and even in those with a disseminated disease. On the other hand, individuals without evolutive candidiasis may carry antibodies (Preisler *et al.*, 1971). Histologic examination by India ink preparation is more reliable: it demonstrates the presence of fungi and the biopsy, in addition, allows its isolation; however, it is not always easy to secure the specimens as there are difficulties depending on the organ to be biopsied or the existence of hemorrhagic risks, especially in leukemic patients.

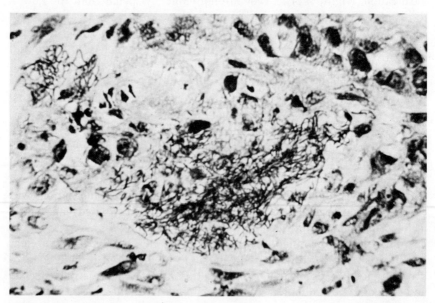

**Fig. 12.**   Micrograph of a bronchial involvement from an esophageal carcinoma; pseudomycelium of *Candida* among neoplastic cells.

## Treatment and Evolution

Therapy of candidiasis of the skin, mouth, or anus may be limited to local action by the application of nystatin or amphotericin pomade, or even of dyes (hexamethyl pararosaniline chloride) on the skin, or by washing the mucous membranes with a suspension of amphotericin or nystatin. These two drugs may also be taken orally in digestive infections, but their efficacy has not been established by controlled trials (Boggs *et al.*, 1961).

Visceral localization, pulmonary in particular, necessitates an intravenous treatment by amphotericin with progressively increasing doses in order to reach 30–50 mg every other day, combined or not with flucytosine (150–200 mg by kg per day), orally or intravenously. Generalized therapy is also needed in serious digestive disorders, such as esophageal candidiasis and ulcerous colon candididasis (Moulinier *et al.*, 1972; Bodey, 1975).

According to Toala *et al.* (1970), the best anticandida agent is amphotericin, active on 90% of the *Candida* isolated at Boston, at the concentration of 0.1 $\mu$g/ml product, while the minimum inhibitory concentration of nystatin on the same specimens is 5 $\mu$g/ml and the sensitivity to flucytosine is even poorer. Moreover, there is a synergistic action between amphotericin B and flucytosine even for a *Candida* resistant to flucytosine alone (Montgomerie *et al.*, 1975). Miconazole may be useful in some cases (Katz and Cassileth, 1977).

The prognosis of these candidiases is generally unfavorable, except for superficial manifestations. The high mortality is due to two reasons: on the one hand, the difficulties of diagnosis lead to an absence or a delay of appropriate therapy; on the other hand, the limits of medical treatment, owing either to the resistance of *Candida* to available drugs, or to the insufficient diffusion of these drugs into the lesions, where the yeasts are embedded and surrounded by an inflammatory and sclerotic reaction (Bodey, 1975).

## ASPERGILLOSIS

### Etiology

*Aspergillus fumigatus* is usually the responsible agent for aspergillosis, but other members of the species may also be observed sporadically: *Aspergillus niger, Asp. versicolor, Asp. clavatus, Asp. glaneus, Asp. flavus, Asp. nidulans*, etc. *Aspergillus* is a saprophyte of the normal subject (Landau *et al.*, 1963). Less frequent than candidiasis, aspergillosis has nevertheless an increasing incidence. Prior to 1950, 1% of the patients in a general hospital population were found to have this infection at necropsy examination compared to 3% in 1963 (Heffermann and Asper, 1966).

In a study by Meyer *et al.* (1973) that dealt with cancer patients, 30 cases of aspergillosis were observed at necropsy examination between 1951 and 1963 and 93 between 1963 and 1973. In addition, in that decade twice as many cases were observed in 1969–1970 as in 1963–1964. This infection is observed in acute leukemias especially, seven times less often in lymphomas, and even more rarely in solid tumors. These figures should nevertheless be compared to the absolute number of leukemias, lymphomas, and solid tumors observed during the same period (Table XXIX).

TABLE XXIX.   Distribution of Aspergillosis According to the Type of Cancer[a]

| Cancer | Number of Cases of Aspergillosis | | |
|---|---|---|---|
| | Localized | Generalized | Total |
| Acute leukemia | 34 | 9 | 43 |
| Chronic leukemia | 7 | 2 | 9 |
| Hodgkin's disease | 6 | 1 | 7 |
| Non-Hodgkin's lymphoma | 13 | 5 | 18 |
| Solid tumor | 9 | 5 | 14 |

[a] From Meyer *et al.* (1973), 1951–1973, National Cancer Institute, Bethesda, Maryland.

Neither age nor sex plays a role in the development of aspergillosis. However, there are many other factors which, regardless of the underlying malignancy, may predispose patients to aspergillosis: a preceding infection caused by *Pseudomonas* is often observed, or a *Pseudomonas* infection is even associated with aspergillosis and it is not possible to affirm whether it is the bacterial infection itself or the antibiotic therapy which favored the development of fungal infection; many patients often receive corticosteroids or cytotoxic chemotherapy or have granulocytopenia (Meyer *et al.*, 1973).

Moreover, aspergillosis is associated with candidiasis in one-third of the cases, with *Pseudomonas* infections in 15% of the cases, and more rarely with other bacterial infections (Meyer *et al.*, 1973).

The lung is almost always involved in aspergillosis (90 out of 93 cases in the series of Meyer *et al.*, 1973) and in 70% of the patients studied it is the only site of infection. Other sites of infection are rarer; in the same series visceral localization was observed only nine times for the heart, brain, and digestive tract, seven for the kidney, five for the liver, four for the thyroid, three for the spleen, and once for the bladder and diaphragm. Skin lesions have been observed by Prystonsky *et al.* (1976). The high percentage of pulmonary aspergillosis is probably explained by respiratory contamination by inhalation of spores. In some cases the portal of entry could be cutaneous (Prystonsky *et al.*, 1976) although these cutaneous lesions might also be hematogenous. At a necropsy, the histologic lesion is often a hemorrhagic infarct of an embolic origin (Wiernick and Serpick, 1969) or is secondary to a pulmonary thrombosis, as *Aspergillus* has a vascular tropism and tends to develop in the lumen of the vessels that it obstructs.

## Clinical Aspects

Aspergillosis almost always causes fever which fails to respond to antibiotic therapy and manifestations related to the localization of the fungi, but the diagnosis is difficult to establish clinically.

Pulmonary infection sometimes presents the aspect of an embolism, with dyspnea, sudden pleuritic chest pain, hemoptysis, and syndrome of localized pulmonary consolidation. Empyemas are rare. Generally the clinical picture is subclinical and the pulmonary localization is discovered by radiography. The image *en grelot* of aspergilloma which is dense inside a light cavity is characteristic but rare in cancer patients (Ramsay and Meyer, 1973). The aspects of bronchopneumonia or localized pneumonias are more frequent. Bronchitis and microabscesses are rare. Outside of the first-mentioned radiologic abnormality, the others are not specific to aspergillosis and may also be observed in cases of phycomycosis and even in candidiasis (Burke and Coltman, 1971).

Other rare localizations are readily latent from the clinical point of view. They cause single or multiple abscesses. Infection of the paranasal sinuses or orbit causes widespread destruction of soft tissues and cartilage of the face. In neurologic aspergillosis, meningeal disorders are rarer than neurologic disorders. Aspergillus provokes single or multiple ulcerations in the mucous membranes of the digestive tract. These ulcerations can be lodged from the esophagus to the rectum and may cause hemorrhages (Meyer *et al.*, 1973). Hepatic infection is presented by abscesses and necrotic zones; it may result in a Budd–Chiari syndrome (Young, 1969). An endocarditis (Kammer and Utz, 1974) and a papillary necrosis (Young *et al.*, 1970) have also been described.

This emphasizes the vasculotropic and thrombogenic character of aspergillosis infection in cancer patients. Multiple embolic localizations are characteristic of aspergillosis in these patients. They are not exceptional (23 out of 93 for Meyer *et al.*, 1973), and may be found either in different sites, or even multiple sites in the lung (Burke and Coltman, 1971). Necrotic cutaneous lesions may be associated with disseminated infection (Bodey, 1975). They are usually ecthyma gangrenosum as in *Pseudomonas* septicemias (Prystonsky *et al.*, 1975). This dissemination appears to be hematogenous, but blood cultures are seldom positive (Meyer *et al.*, 1973). These symptoms are very different from the manifestation of aspergillosis in noncancerous patients, who present only pulmonary infection.

## Diagnosis

Diagnosis is particularly difficult except for the cases presenting typical pulmonary lesions on the x-ray. Cultures are positive in only one-third of the patients; in addition, the fact that Meyer *et al.* (1973). have never isolated *Aspergillus* from the blood, spinal fluid, or urine of their 93 patients should be kept in mind. Also, the *Aspergillus* present in sputum may simply be saprophytic (Meyer *et al.*, 1973). The detection of antibodies is possible, but falls short of the mark, especially for disseminated aspergillosis in leukemias and lymphomas (Young and Bennett, 1971). Bronchial brushing with aspiration and pulmonary biopsy, when they may be done, aid in establishing the diagnosis.

One of the reasons for the poor prognosis of aspergillosis is that the diagnosis is seldom established while the patient is alive. Dissemination is directly responsible for death in 45% of the cases (Meyer *et al.*, 1973).

A systematic search for antibodies by an immunodiffusion test was performed during 1 year in 80 leukemic patients (Schaeffer *et al.*, 1976): 12 serologic conversions were observed and in 6 patients further isolation of *Aspergillus* confirmed the diagnosis; 4 out of these 6 patients were cured owing to an early treatment; nevertheless, 3 patients remained seronegative in spite of *Aspergillus* isolation.

## Treatment and Evolution

The treatment is chiefly amphotericin B; flucytosine is active on only 30% of the *Aspergillus*. Since the majority of infections are diagnosed at necropsy, experience with any therapy has been limited. However, pulmonary aspergillosis has been cured by amphotericin B administered systematically associated with nystatin in aerosol (Vedder and Scharr, 1969; Burke and Coltman, 1971), by amphotericin B alone (Pennington, 1976), or by amphotericin associated with granulocyte transfusions (Gergovich *et al.*, 1975). Sometimes, surgical cures may be useful. The remission of the underlying cancer (in particular leukemia) is a favorable element, but not obligatory, for the efficacy of the treatment (Meyer *et al.*, 1973).

## OTHER FUNGAL INFECTIONS

### Cryptococcosis

*Cryptococcus neoformans,* a saprophyte in animals (particularly in the pigeon), enters via the respiratory tract, where it provokes symptoms of a banal pneumonia, then tends to spread to the nervous system (Selz and Novotny, 1976), and even disseminates.

This fungal infection is well known in France; more than half of the cases are observed in immunosuppressed patients. Only 3% of patients with primary pulmonary infection have cancer and 15% of patients with an underlying malignancy have meningitis. Almost all patients with disseminated cryptococcosis have malignant diseases (Siguier *et al.,* 1970; Roujeau *et al.,* 1971; Lewis and Rabinovich, 1972). Patients with lymphomas and leukemias are more often affected than those with solid tumors.

Pulmonary infection provokes a subacute or chronic pneumonia with cough, pleuritic pain, fever, weight loss. X-Ray examination shows various manifestations: nodular, miliary, or sometimes cavitary lesions (Campbell, 1966).

Neuromeningeal infection may be insidious at the onset and may be confused with lymphomatous involvement of the meninges. The meningeal syndrome is more or less clinically evident (Leng *et al.,* 1974). The cerebrospinal fluid is usually hypertensive with increased protein concentration, decreased glucose concentration, and lymphocytosis, but, in some patients, may be normal. *Cryptococcus* can be seen by direct examination of cerebrospinal fluid with India ink in 60% of the patients; it can be cultured on Sabouraud's medium; it may also be detected by specific serum antibodies (Kaufman and Blumer, 1968).

The disseminated disease may infect the lung, central nervous system, heart, spleen, pancreas, adrenals, kidneys, skin, and bone. Cutaneous lesions may be acneiform, nodular, or ulcerated (Bodey, 1975).

If cryptococcal meningitis is easy to identify, it is not so for other localizations. These may necessitate histologic examination of the skin, lung, or serologic reactions, which search for either cryptococcal antigens in the serum, in the cerebrospinal fluid by specific serums, or anticryptococcal antibodies by agglutination or indirect immunofluorescence (Levine *et al.,* 1972).

*Cryptococcus* is usually sensitive to amphotericin and flucytosine. The efficacy of these therapies given intravenously or, in the case of cryptococcal meningitis intrathecally, is relative (Utz *et al.,* 1975). The underlying malignancy and corticosteroid therapy usually condition the poor prognosis (Diamond and Bennett, 1974), although the appearance of acquired fungal resistance under treatment has also been described (Fass and Perkins, 1971). The mortality rate for disseminated cryptococcosis is 80% (Lewis and Rabinovich, 1972).

## Mucormycosis

The responsible agents are phycomycetes of the group mucorales, represented by *Rhizopus, Absidia,* and *Mucor.* These fungal infections are observed especially in the United States, where, like other fungal infections, they are mainly observed in patients with leukemias and lymphomas. In a series of 47 cases, 32 occurred in patients with leukemia, 8 in patients with malignant lymphoma, and 3 in patients with multiple myeloma (Meyer *et al.,* 1973). These authors emphasize that the mucormycosis caused infection in 2% of patients with leukemia in 1962, whereas they caused infections in 8% of the same type of patients in 1971.

These fungi cause different clinical symptoms in cancer patients and in patients suffering other illnesses, in particular diabetes. In diabetics they usually cause a sinusitis with orbital cellulitis, whereas in cancer patients they tend to generalize and provoke pulmonary, digestive, or cutaneous manifestations (Meyer *et al.,* 1973) or to disseminate and fail to give any specific symptoms; hence their origin may be unrecognized.

The diagnosis is mainly based on histologic examination of involved tissues and fungal cultures taken from these sites. The physiopathologic process of this fungal infection resembles that of aspergillosis: tendency to vascular invasion, with resultant thrombosis and infarction. Mucormycosis is thus difficult to identify clinically (Bartrum *et al.,* 1973; Medoff and Kobayashi, 1972; Kwan-Chung *et al.,* 1975). For the present there are no reliable serologic tests.

The treatment is amphotericin and flucytosine; an oral administration of a saturated solution of potassium iodide may be indicated (Bennett, 1974).

## Histoplasmosis

These are also fungal infections found mainly in the United States. In the general population, *Histoplasma capsulatum* causes either an inapparent infection or a chronic or acute bronchopneumonia (Sarosi *et al.,* 1971). In cancer patients, and in particular malignant blood diseases, *Histoplasma* like other fungi tends to disseminate from the lungs to the liver and to the nervous system (Cox and Hughes, 1974).

The lack of specific clinical manifestations does not facilitate its identification, but bone marrow culture done on a patient with fever and with or without pulmonary symptoms, permits the diagnosis, as does the culture or histologic examination of tissue lesions (Hughes, 1971). Specific antibodies may be found.

Histoplasma is sensitive to amphotericin B and can be efficaciously treated (Cox and Hughes, 1974).

## Other Fungi

Other fungi may be observed: geotrichosis (Chang and Buerger, 1964), blastomycosis, chromoblastomycosis, coccidioidomycosis, and infections caused by *Torulopsis* and *Rhodorula* (Louria et al., 1967). Their frequency in cancer patients does not seem to be increasing in spite of the prolonged survival of these patients and immunosuppressive therapy (Levine et al., 1972).

Out of 44 coccidioidomycoses, recently collected by Deresinski and Stevens (1974), 13 cases were observed in immunosuppressed patients among whom 8 had malignant lymphoma, 1 had myeloma, and 1 had myxosarcoma. This mycosis seems to be favored by chemotherapy more than by radiotherapy of the cancer itself. In comparison with healthy fungal carriers, fungal infection is rare, usually pulmonary. Its onset is usually very rapid with an appearance of pulmonary lesions within 24 hr. Septicemic and metastatic dissemination is frequent in such patients, whereas it is observed only in 1% of other patients. This dissemination is enhanced by lymphopenia. Diagnosis may be affirmed during lifetime by serologic tests, but is usually established only by necropsy. Generalized forms are almost always lethal.

The frequency of the infections caused by *Torulopsis glabrata* in cancer patients has been also recently underlined (Aisner et al., 1974; Rivera and Cangir, 1975; Aisner et al., 1976; Valdivieso et al., 1976). The percentage of carriers seems to be steady but the number of infections is increasing; the main localizations are pulmonary, esophageal, or renal and some septicemias are observed. Frequently this mycosis is associated with another fungal infection (aspergillosis, candidiasis). Diagnosis is made in only 10% of the patients before death. Actually the mortality is high; it is due to *Torulopsis* in half of the cases and to an advanced cancer in other patients.

# CHAPTER 8

# Parasitic Infections

Parasitic infections observed in cancer patients are dominated by two discernibly different affections: toxoplasmosis and pneumocystosis. Toxoplasmosis, well represented in France, causes a variety of pathologic manifestations, depending on the patients and on the involved organs. On the other hand, pneumocystosis practically only gives a pneumonic infection and only in compromised patients. The diagnosis of toxoplasmosis is determined by serologic investigations, which give results that are not always easy to interpret, while the diagnosis of pneumocystosis is based on demonstration of the presence of parasites. In the two cases, latent infestation appears to be more frequent than the acute parasitic disease.

## TOXOPLASMOSIS

*Toxoplasma gondii* is a ubiquitous protozoa and an obligate intracellular parasite. In humans it may be responsible for congenital disease or acquired affection. Acquired toxoplasmosis in a healthy person is generally inapparent or benign. However, it can cause severe disease in patients with underlying malignancies or in patients receiving immunosuppressive treatment (Gleason and Hamlin, 1974). Such is the case in cancer patients, or at least some of them (Chauvergne *et al.*, 1969).

### Etiology

In summing the cases collected by Vietzke *et al.*, (1968) and those published since then about 50 observations can be collated in which malignant blood diseases, especially Hodgkin's disease which represents half of the total, dominate (Table XXX). These cancer patients are characterized by a deficit of cell-mediated or humoral immune response, and/or are receiving corticosteroids or heavy and immunosuppressive chemotherapy (see Chapter 3). They comprise an independent distribution of age and a slight masculine predominance.

The origin of this parasitic infection may be a reactivation of a latent congenital toxoplasmosis, as seen in some where the sequella of such an

TABLE XXX.   Reviews of Toxoplasmosis in Cancer Patients

| References | Leukemias | | Lymphomas | | Solid Tumors |
|---|---|---|---|---|---|
| | Acute | Chronic | Hodgkin's | Non-Hodgkin's | |
| Bernard et al. (1962) | 1 | | | | |
| Lemaire et al. (1965) | 1 | | | | |
| Cassi and Visca (1966) | | | 1 | | |
| Vietzke et al. (1968)[a] | 4 | 3 | 8 | 2 | 2 |
| Abell and Holland (1969) | 1 | | | | |
| Barlotta et al. (1969) | | | 2 | | |
| Lunde et al. (1970) | 1 | 1 | | | |
| Luna and Lichtinger (1971) | | | 1 | | |
| Neu (1971) | | 1 | 1 | | |
| Roth et al. (1971) | 1 | | | | |
| Siegel et al. (1971) | 4 | | | | |
| Carey et al. (1973) | | 3 | 9 | 1 | 1 |
| Gleason and Halmin (1974) | | | 1 | | 1 |
| Wuttke (1974) | | | 1 | | |
| Masson et al. (1975) | | 1 | 1 | | |
| Beauvais et al. (1976) | 1 | | | | |
| Personal cases | | | 2 | 1 | |
| Total | 13 | 10 | 27 | 4 | 4 |

[a] Personal cases and review.

infection persist. It may also be a newly acquired infection transmitted in the usual ways, especially by the ingestion of improperly cooked meat containing cysts or by contact with cats. The transmission by leukocytic concentrates from donors with chronic myeloid leukemia has been described (Roth et al., 1971; Siegel et al., 1971; Beauvais et al., 1976).

## Clinical Aspects

In a healthy individual, toxoplasmosis is either inapparent or causes minor manifestations and has a benign evolution; however, in cancer patients the protozoa cause severe diseases with a marked general syndrome and localized manifestations. The general syndrome consists of fever and generalized erythema. The fever may be very high, without detectable infectious foci; the blood cultures are persistently negative (although there is an associated bacterial septicemia in some cases); broad spectrum antibiotic therapy remains ineffective.

Infection of the central nervous system is one of the most frequent manifestations and is reported in more than half of the cases. At the onset of the disease there may be confusion with disorientation and headache; and the cerebrospinal fluid is only slightly modified. Encephalitis is more serious and most often diffuse; the onset is by syncope and is followed by a coma, more or less deep, sometimes accompanied by vomiting. Localized neurologic symptoms are rare: hemiparesia, cranial nerve palsies, amaurosis. There is no associated chorioretinitis (Vietzke et al., 1968; Townsend et al., 1975). However, in two Hodgkin's patients we have observed an isolated chorioretinitis, without an associated general syndrome, corresponding in one case to a newly acquired infection and in the other to a reactivation of toxoplasmosis (Hoerni et al., 1977; Fig. 13).

Pleuropulmonary infections, mainly pneumonia, causing respiratory distress and eventually death, are also frequent, as well as myocardial infections which may cause an irreversible cardiac insufficiency.

Lymph-node localization, frequent in healthy individuals, is, on the contrary, rare and often misleading in patients with malignant lymphoma, although the size of toxoplasmic lymph nodes is always small. Any other sort of disorder may rarely predominate, for example, an acute pancreatitis (Roth et al., 1971).

Generally, these diverse manifestations are associated and constitute a severe disease with a rapidly fatal evolution. An extension of the neoplastic process may be suspected, but these neurologic syndromes, which

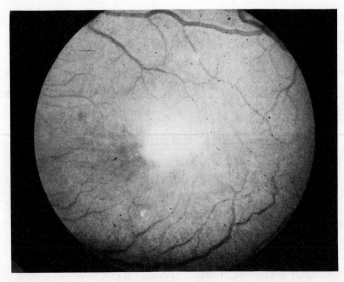

**Fig. 13.** Exudative lesion on the left macula due to an acquired toxoplasm in a 47-year-old woman with Hodgkin's disease.

are rare in Hodgkin's disease, should raise suspicion of an intercurrent especially infectious complication.

Moreover, it is not rare that toxoplasmosis is associated with another infection, bacterial, viral (herpes, cytomegalic inclusions disease) (Vietzke *et al.*, 1968; Luna and Lichtinger, 1971; Gleason and Hamlin, 1974), or parasitic (pneumocystosis) (Gleason and Hamlin, 1974).

### Diagnosis

Toxoplasmosis should be suspected in these various circumstances and confirmed by appropriate examinations. A lymphadenopathy should sometimes be biopsied when it does not seem to mesh (either by its chronology, context, or aspect) with the diagnosis of the underlying malignancy. The histologic aspects of lymph-node infection by toxoplasmosis are now well known and should be easily distinguished from those of lymphoma and Hodgkin's disease particularly (Dorfman and Remingron, 1973).

Serologic tests are necessary, but their results are sometimes difficult to interpret. In patients with clinical manifestations corresponding to toxoplasmosis, serologic tests give decisive arguments in favor of that diagnosis (Lunde *et al.*, 1970). A significant rise in titer of a serological test from an earlier test at the time of diagnosis of cancer (serologic tests should be systematically performed in all Hodgkin's patients) is an indisputable argument in favor of a recently acquired infection. With a low baseline antibody titer, an important increase in antibody titer affirms a reactivation of the protozoa. If an initial serologic investigation has not been done, a very high antibody titer is in favor of a toxoplasmosis; an increase in only IgM antibodies affirms a recent infection.

In patients without particular symptoms of toxoplasmosis, systematic and repeated serologic testing may demonstrate important variations in the antibodies' titer. Our experience with the lytic test of toxoplasma (Chauvergne *et al.*, 1969) approaches that of Lunde *et al.* (1970) with a variety of serologic tests: together with the apparent disease (accompanied by clinical symptoms and convergent serologic modification), there are also frequent positive conversions or important increases in antibody titer without any clinical symptoms. When there is a serologic conversion, an inapparent clinical infection may be affirmed. When there is no serologic baseline (owing to lack of initial serologic testing) or in patients who were  only weakly positive in the beginning, it is not possible to determine if the increase in antibody titer corresponds either to an infraclinical reactivation of toxoplasma or to a nonspecific increase of immunoglobulins, which accompanies the hematologic malignancy.

Regardless of the exact reason for the increase of this antibody titer, it is observed in spite of the immunosuppression presented by these patients, since this immune deficiency especially concerns cell-mediated immune response: in a Hodgkin's patient who presented a high positivity of the dye test, the intradermal test to toxoplasmine was negative.

Actually, the diagnosis of toxoplasmosis can be completely confirmed only if there are clinical symptoms combined with serologic modifications, and also often necropsied results which are positive for this protozoa. This explains numerous publications which report indisputable observations with necropsy data. For several of them, however, the diagnosis of toxoplasmosis has been established only postmortem.

Histologic examination schematically demonstrates two types of isolated or associated modifications; on the one hand, the protozoa may be seen as intracellular pseudocysts; on the other hand, there are inflammatory lesions. The brain, lung, and heart are the most infested organs (Gleason and Hamlin, 1974). In the brain, the typical lesion, which may involve the hypophysis, associates small foci of microglial cells and mononucleated inflammatory cells along with dispersed necrotic foci in the white and gray matter. In the lung a diffuse interstitial pneumonia with hyaline membranes and thinned alveolar septa infiltrated with round cells is observed. In the myocardium scattered inflammatory and necrotic foci are found. Electron microscopy may be interesting, especially for the morphologic study of toxoplasma (Luna and Lichtinger, 1971).

## Treatment and Evolution

The evolution is often unfavorable in the published observations owing to the failure of diagnosis, the severity of toxoplasmosis (in particular in case of neurologic infection), and the associated cancer.

If the diagnosis is established early enough, treatment (owing to the usual severity of the disease) may be administered: spiramycin and pyrimethanin, sulfonamides or cotrimoxazole; however, the hematologic toxicity of pyrimethanin often limits its use. Relapses are possible (Roth et al., 1971).

## PNEUMOCYTOSIS

Identified in 1909 by Chagas, *Pneumocystis carinii* is a microorganism which is not definitely classified, but is probably a protozoa; it is ubiquitous in men and animals and has worldwide distribution. It mainly causes pneumonia via the respiratory tract, but sometimes causes disseminated infections, particularly with lymph-node and splenic infections (Barnett et al. 1969).

## Etiology

Pneumocytis is a pathogenic agent which is almost only opportunistic since it causes disease only in compromised patients. (Ruskin and Remington (1967) dedicated their first article in their series studying opportunistic infection to *Pneumocystis*.) Leukemic patients, especially children, suffer the most from this infection; they represent two-thirds of cancer patients with parasitic infections, but other hematologic malignancies may be involved (Tables VII, X, and XXXI). In these cancer patients pneumocystosis causes nearly half of the confirmed interstitial pneumonias, far ahead of aspergillosis, cytomegalic inclusion disease, cryptococcosis, and toxoplasmosis (Goodell *et al.*, 1970).

Some authors think that pneumocystosis is an infection of recent years (Fischer *et al.*, 1969), but actually it has been established that infestation, found in 5% of adults with malignant blood diseases (Esterly, 1968) or of children with cancer (Sedaghatian and Singer, 1972) and judged on systematic necropsies, has been stable for the last 20 years; however, the frequency of clinical pneumocystosis is definitely increasing.

TABLE XXXI.  Reviews of Pneumocystosis in Cancer Patients

| | Leukemias | | Lymphomas | | |
|---|---|---|---|---|---|
| References | Acute | Chronic | Hodgkin's | Non-Hodgkin's | Solid Tumors |
| Hendry and Patrick (1962) | 5 | 3 | | 2 | |
| Nathorst-Windahl *et al.* (1964) | 1 | 1 | | | |
| Esterly and Warner (1965) | 6 | 1 | 2 | 3 | |
| Callerame and Nadel (1966) | | 2 | | | |
| Ruskin and Remington (1967) | | 1 | 1 | 1 | |
| Smith and Gaspar (1968) | | 1 | | | |
| Brazinsky and Phillips (1969) | | | 1 | 1 | |
| DeVita *et al.* (1969) | 1 | | | 1 | |
| Einzig *et al.* (1969) | 1 | | | | |
| Fischer *et al.* (1969) | 1 | 1 | 1 | | |
| Kennedy *et al.* (1970) | 1 | | | | |
| Forrest (1972) | 2 | 2 | 2 | 1 | 1 |
| Rosen *et al.* (1972) | 2 | 3 | 6 | 6 | 3 |
| Sedaghatian and Singer (1972) | 9 | | 1 | 4 | 1 |
| Hughes *et al.* (1973) | 45 | | 1 | 2 | 3 |
| Drew *et al.* (1974) | | 1 | | 1 | |
| Pujet *et al.* (1974) | | | | 1 | |
| Singer *et al.* (1975) | 6 | | 4 | | 1 |
| Total | 80 | 16 | 19 | 23 | 9 |

This increase has been linked to the particularly intensive treatments given to cancer patients in these last 12 years (Perera *et al.*, 1970).

. Hence it seems likely that there are healthy carriers, perhaps among the medical staff, who may transmit the parasite, but in most cases, the infection is due to the activation of a preexisting latent infestation. Infected patients should be isolated owing to the possibility of cross-infection (Ruskin and Remington, 1967; Brazinsky and Phillips, 1969) or transmission by hospital staff (Singer *et al.*, 1975).

Infection goes through three stages: inhalation of the parasite, probably in C form; proliferation in the cytoplasm of macrophages of the alveolar walls and desquamation of these cells in the alveolar cavity; and finally, aggravation of the intricated processes of macrophagy, proliferation, and desquamation is responsible for the appearance of clinical manifestations (Hughes *et al.*, 1973).

## Clinical Aspects

The disease may develop slowly or rapidly: at the onset tachypnea is generally observed only when the patient produces an effort, but progressively it becomes constant, with an evident respiratory insufficiency. It is accompanied by a cyanosis of increasing intensity (which a functional investigation may link to a hypoxia with hypocapnia caused by alveolar capillary block) and a rarely productive dry cough. Fever is generally absent in the child, but present in the adult (Bientz and Rochemaure, 1973).

Physical findings are usually minimal. Sometimes there are some crepitant rales or a hypersonority linked to a compensating emphysema. Thus x-rays are essential.

## Radiology

Pneumocystosis typically causes a diffuse and bilateral pneumonia: a patchy reticulogranular process evolves toward the formation of more extensive nonsystematized infiltrates, which are most prominent in the peri-hilar region and spare the periphery of the parenchyma, at least in the beginning (Fig. 14) (Forrest, 1972). However, atypical images may also be observed: asymmetric, even unilateral, lesions, lobar localization, and moderate or large pleural effusion. The frequency of these manifestations in (17 out of 30 observations of Doppmann *et al.*, 1975) demonstrates that the treatment cannot be based on these findings. More typical images might arouse suspicion of pneumocystosis, but are not specific enough to confirm the diagnosis and may be difficult to distinguish from other pneumonias, leukemic infiltrates, or lymphomatous metastasis or even chemotherapeutic fibrosis.

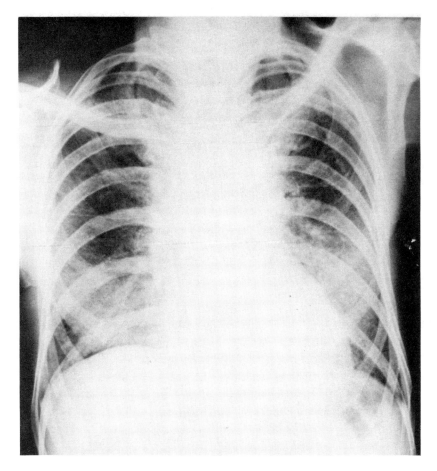

**Fig. 14.** Typical x-ray picture of pulmonary pneumocystosis in a patient with malignant histiocytosis.

## Diagnosis

This parasite has not yet been cultivated, thus it has to be patiently and attentively searched for by a variety of histopathological techniques.

Sputum examinations have yielded practically nothing. Bronchial secretions taken directly by bronchoscopy (Fortuny *et al.*, 1970) or by transtracheal puncture (Lau *et al.*, 1976) are seldom positive. Bronchopulmonary washings give more abundant and richer material (Drew *et al.*, 1974). Generally, more important specimens are required: transbronchial or transparietal pulmonary punctures (De Vita *et al.*, 1969; Johnson and Johnson, 1970; Hughes *et al.*, 1973) or pulmonary biopsy by surgery or bronchoscopy. All these procedures are difficult when marked respiratory insufficiency or coagulation defects exist, which is the case in the majority of the patients.

Hence, the endobronchial brush biopsy, an examination which is easy to perform and is without danger, affirms the diagnosis in a little more than half of the cases. It gives interesting results if it is done strictly according to approved technique, with perfectly adapted material and competent personnel (Kernec et al., 1974).

Smears should be made from aspirates and fixed by either air drying or alcohol–ether. There are various stains, particularly those using a silver preparation, which demonstrate the parasites, generally in form of cysts, round, bracketlike or comma shaped, containing eight punctuations typically arranged in a rosette.

Histologic examination shows pneumonia with thickening of the interalveolar separations, presence of a foamy exudate (beehive aspect) in the alveoli, and cysts which stain with PAS and silver (Esterly and Warner, 1965).

Even though specimens are collected and processed correctly, the parasite is seldom observed and diagnosis is only definitely affirmed by pulmonary specimens taken at necropsy, when this is possible. Serologic tests have been studied, but for the moment do not give conclusive results. Until now indirect immunofluorescence tests have not given reliable results (Arnaud et al., 1976).

## Treamtent and Evolution

During the last few years, pentamidine has been the most active drug against this parasite. It is administered intramuscularly, at 4 mg/kg per day over a period of 12–14 days, and strictly surveyed. More than half of the patients recover (Johnson and Johnson, 1970). However, some pneumocystoses are not sensitive to this treatment and some patients present important adverse reactions (azotemia, hypoglycemia, hypotension, liver function abnormalities, and necrosis at injection sites) that lead to the discontinuation of the treatment; a case of severe thrombocytopenia has also been related to this drug (Levy et al., 1974). Presently trimethoprim-sulfamethoxazole (cotrimoxazole) is more frequently used because it has a similar efficacy and is much less toxic (Lau and Young, 1976). The dosages used vary between 960 and 1200 mg trimethoprim and 4800 and 6000 mg of sulfamethoxazole per day in three or four oral or intravenous administrations. Since this drug is well tolerated, patients with suspected pneumocystosis may be treated even if the diagnosis has not been absolutely confirmed.

The evolution of the disease is still unfavorable and terminates fatally in a few weeks for more than half of the patients because the diagnosis is not established or the treatment is not efficacious. A few spontaneous recoveries have been reported, but there is a possibility of relapse after a temporary favorable evolution depending on the nature of the cancer and the treatment it necessitates (Hughes *et al.*, 1973).

## OTHER PARASITOSES

A variety of parasitosis, such as taeniasis or trichmoniasis, may be observed in cancer patients, but they have neither a particular incidence nor special characteristics. Masur *et al.* (1976) isolated a *Trichomonas* from a meningitis along with *Streptococcus, Eikenella corrodens*, and *Bacillus fragilis* in one patient with an esophageal carcinoma which had been treated by radiotherapy. We have incidentally discovered microfilaria in two patients with malignant lymphoma, in one by leukoconcentration and in the other in a spleen specimen after splenectomy.

Infections with *Strongyloides* are quite different. The first cases were published by Rogers and Nelson (1966) and since then 15 other observations have been reported (Table XXXII).

*Strongyloides stercoralis*, a helminth, may be carried several years, or even many decades, in a latent phase in individuals who have left an endemic area (mainly Southeast Asia, Equatorial Africa, South America, the West Indies, but also the United States and Europe). It may cause an infection and can cause severe or even fatal disease by the diffuse development of larvas in the colon, lungs, liver, and other organs. This development may be favored by impairing intestinal transit or lesions of the intestinal mucous membrane (Purtillo *et al.*, 1974).

This parasitosis mainly causes digestive disorders (epigastric pain, nausea, vomiting, diarrhea, ileus), weight loss, dehydration, edemas, and more rarely dyspnea.

TABLE XXXII. Reviews of Strongylodiasis in Cancer Patients

| References | Leukemias | | Lymphomas | | Solid Tumors |
|---|---|---|---|---|---|
| | Acute | Chronic | Hodgkin's | Non-Hodgkin's | |
| Rogers and Nelson (1966) | | 1 | 1 | | |
| Yim *et al.* (1970) | | | 1 | | |
| Rivera *et al.* (1970) | 3 | | 1 | 2 | |
| Adam *et al.* (1973) | | | 2 | 1 | |
| Purtillo *et al.* (1974) | | 1 | | 1 | 3 |
| Total | 3 | 2 | 5 | 4 | 3 |

Eosinophilia is not constant, probably because of the associated immune deficiency. The larvas of the parasite may be found in stool and urine if a careful examination is performed. Strongyloidiasis may be associated with another parasitic digestive disease, or even with bacterial or fungal infections. At necropsy, eggs, larvas, and adult forms are found in the ileal crypts, the walls of the colon are edematous and fibrosed, and the mucous membrane presents clearly defined ulcers. The insufficiency of delayed hyeprsensitivity is demonstrated by the lack of granulomatous reactions to the contact of the larvas. The parasite is seldom observed in the liver (involved via the portal vein), lungs, spleen, heart, subcutaneous tissues, and lymph nodes.

If the diagnosis is established early enough, the patient may be treated by thiabendazole administered orally at the dose of 25 mg/kg, twice daily for 3–4 days.

The frequency of the latent parasitic infestation in some individuals justifies routine studies; its eradication should be achieved prior to chemotherapy for the cancer.

Two cases of transfusional malaria were observed by Tapper and Armstrong (1976): in one patient with acute myeloid leukemia the evolution was benign; in the other patient, who had been splenectomized and had an advanced colon carcinoma, the malaria symptoms were malignant but the evolution was favorable with specific treatment.

Relations between liver cancers and schistosomiasis are quite different (Nakashima et al., 1975). Schistosoma japonicum does not superinfect patients with cancer but seems to play an etiologic role at the beginning of the cancer, along with other factors, just as some aforementioned viruses (see Chapter 6).

# 3

## Treatment and Evolution

CHAPTER 9

# Preventive Treatment

Since most infections observed in cancer patients depend directly or indirectly on paraneoplastic immune deficiency, owing to the cancer, the most important prophylactic treatment of these infections is the anticancer treatment itself. We shall only consider the main points of this treatment, concentrating on the aspects which are especially interesting for infections. Then, we shall discuss various anti-infectious means which are also useful and are more directly related to our subject, but not necessarily more important in everyday practice.

The useful measures generally depend on the pathophysiology (Chapter 3) and the factors which favor infection (Chapter 2) in cancer patients (Table XXXIII).

## ANTICANCER TREATMENT

Regardless of the type of treatment, intervention is either direct by causing the disappearance or, at least, the regression of the neoplastic lesion which favored a local infection, or indirect by improving the general status, and in particular, the immunologic condition of the patient. Moreover, a variety of means reduces their infectious hazards.

### Direct Influence

The regression of tumoral lesions under the influence of treatment often corresponds to a decrease in the infectious risks or may even prevent their occurrence. For example, epithelial lesions, which constitute a break in the skin or mucous membranes, provide both a local infectious focus and a potential portal of entry. Their healing by either radiotherapy, surgical removal, or the reduction of deep lesions before they have destroyed the primary barriers is the means of eliminating or reducing the risks of superinfection. The same is true for compressive tumors which favor an infection beyond the stenosis that they provoke. The control, or even better, the suppression of the tumor, removes the cause of the stenosis, reestablishes a normal, or at least a more satisfying, drainage, and thus reduces the risks of retention and superinfection.

TABLE XXXIII.   Schematic Representation of Preventive Treatments
in Cancer Patients

| Factors Favoring Infections (See Table XI) | Preventive Treatments |
|---|---|
| Tumor | Anticancer Treatments |
|   Local disorders |   Radiotherapy–surgery–chemotherapy |
|     Ulceration |     Curative |
|     Stenosis and retention |     Palliative |
|   Systemic consequences |   Rehabilitation |
|     Decubitis | |
|     Malnutrition | |
|     Immunologic deficiency | |
| Medical Actions | |
|   Hospitalization |   Hospital hygiene |
|   Investigations |   Restriction of hospitalization and investigations |
|   Cancer treatments | |
|     Radiotherapy |   Preservation of epithelium |
|     Surgery |   Discontinued chemotherapy |
|     Chemotherapy | |
|     Immunotherapy | |
|   Adjuvant treatments | |
|     Antibiotics |   Reduction of corticosteroids |
|     Others |   Local disinfection |
| |   Vaccinations |
| |   Prophylactic antibiotics |
| |   Isolation |

Associated with hemorrhagic or esthetic inconveniences, an infectious risk may be considered as an indication for a "cleaning act" which eliminates a locally ulcerated or functionally bothersome lesion, even if this localized treatment does not offer any prolongation of survival in a generalized cancer. These interventions are not always satisfying: ureters diverted because of neoplastic stenosis of a prostatic or uterine origin may eliminate the risks of infection above the stenosis but add other risks linked to the nonphysiologic anastomosis of the ureters. Thus, only the main lines of approach may be indicated, as each case must be studied individually.

### Indirect Influence

Control of neoplastic evolution has evidently a very favorable influence. Both general deterioration and infections depending on localized lesions or on metabolic and general immunologic deficiency can be avoided. Curing the cancer prevents severe infections which occur during the terminal evolution for half of the cancer patients who die.

Vertebral or pelvic–femoral metastasis should be carefully looked for and treated generally by radiotherapy to avoid long bedridden periods which add additional infectious risks to already existing unfavorable conditions.

The regression of paraneoplastic immune deficiency is not immediately perceived. The considerable improvement in the prognosis of Hodgkin's disease, particularly predisposed to superinfections, has hardly modified the development of banal infections such as herpes zoster, but has considerably reduced the number of severe infections, such as complicated herpes zoster, which are the consequences of evolutive and advanced diseases which, in most cases, are fatal. Immunologic insufficiency, which is linked to the disease, regresses after efficacious treatment and complete remission. The minimal immunologic deficiency remaining in some patients who are in remission for several years and probably cured is difficult to interpret if a precise evaluation has not been done prior to any pathologic symptoms. For some patients it is an initial state eventually favoring the appearance of the malignancy (Chapter 2), while for others it is a consequence of the treatment, particularly of widespread lymph-node irradiation (Crowther, 1973).

The evolution of paraneoplastic immunologic insufficiency has been followed very precisely in multiple myelomas by the quantitative measurement of immunoglobulins. If the chemothrapy is efficacious and reduces both the tumoral population and the level of pathologic immunoglobulins, the decrease in normal immunoglobulins is corrected (Sullivan and Salmon, 1972). Although an exact correlation has not yet been established, it can be deduced that the infectious risks that are dependent on the hypogammaglobulinemia are reduced. This would seem to confirm current clinical experiences.

## Adaptation of Anticancer Treatment

Knowing the risks of infection to which cancer patients are exposed, the medical staff should reduce supplementary infectious risks which depend on the treatment, but maintain an optimal anticancer treatment.

The surgeon should apply the maximum precautions of aseptic technique. Radiotherapy should avoid marked skin reactions and the range of dosage should be altered accordingly.

The medical oncologist, who is most likely to administer severely immunosuppressive therapy, should give preference to discontinuous application of anticancer drugs. This type of therapy respects the immunologic defenses of the patient better than continuous treatment does (Amiel et al., 1967; Mathé et al., 1969). Hence, it may be observed and appreciated that one of the last cancers treated by continuous chemotherapy, chronic lymphoid leukemia, is now treated discontinuously. This treatment seems to be just as efficacious and certainly avoids aggravating spontaneous marked immunologic insufficiency in this affection (Knospe et al., 1974; Hoerni-Simon et al., 1977). Presently research has been undertaken to realize immunologic restoration by utilizing transfer factor; however, the employed means do not give complete satisfaction (Khan et al., 1975). In all cases granulocytosis is regularly and carefully surveyed and treatment is interrupted or reduced if there is neutropenia, even though peripheral neutropenia is only indicative and sometimes unreliable evidence and does not necessarily reflect the neutrophil stock of the patient's reserves (Deinard et al., 1974).

Discontinuance of prolonged treatment with corticosteroids (which have no anticancer effect, except in lymphoid cancers) and thus avoidance of its constant immunosuppressive effect is progress; one should not, however, overlook certain circumstances in which these drugs are useful.

However, these precautions cannot always be respected and in order to treat some cancers correctly, or to offer better chances of recovery, it is sometimes necessary to apply treatments which indisputably favor superinfections. Thus, an acute lymphoid leukemia must be treated by corticosteroids for a relatively prolonged period and other acute leukemias must be placed in bone marrow aplasia in order to obtain a complete remission. In these cases anti-infectious treatments are very important.

## ANTI-INFECTIOUS TREATMENTS

Anti-infectious treatments should not be reserved only for exceptional cases. However, since the majority of cancer patients do not have major infectious problems, simple but rigorous anti-infectious measures are often sufficient. Exceptional treatments for certain patients or particular cancers are seldom needed.

### General Anti-Infectious Measures

These are the simplest and most important for the majority of cancer patients. These patients benefit from the improvement of general sanitary measures. For example, these measures explain the reduction of tuberculosis in cancer subjects, as also in the general population (Kaplan et al., 1974). In most cases, these measures are the same precautions that are taken for any patient and in all hospital services, but when cancer patients and cancer services are involved, these measures must be attentively surveyed.

Hospitalization of cancer patients should be avoided whenever possible; home care or outpatient service is preferable and avoids the hazards of contamination inherent to any collectivity, hospitals in particular. When it is necessary it should be reduced to a strict minimum.

We cannot detail all the numerous efficacious measures for correct hospital hygiene: the methods concerning disinfection of wards, clothing of the medical staff, laundry, and food. Routine periodic cultures reveal the microbial ecology in a given hospital service. Patients should be isolated: wards should be replaced by rooms which lodge two or three patients, if individual rooms are not always available. These patients need to be protected from all types of contamination (medical staff, visitors, flowers). If possible, patients with the same type of illness should not be concentrated in only one hospital unit.

For hospitalized patients the most basic hygienic care must be employed. This care can be reinforced for certain susceptible patients, such as those with leukemia. Complete bed care should be given and special attention should be given to the scalp and natural orifices such as ears, nose, anus, or vagina—solutions of hexachlorophene, betadine, or quaternary ammonia are recommended and special disinfectant shampoos should be used. These cleaning methods are not aimed at sterilizing patients but rather to eliminate certain microorganisms from their endogenous flora (particularly the Gram-negative bacilli) which may later cause a severe infection. If an evident infectious focus exists in a leukemic patient, and his specific cancer treatment is not very urgent, it is better to first eliminate the infection, for if the patient is placed in bone marrow aplasia, the infection might become extremely severe.

Dental examination and consequent care are imperative, especially in patients receiving cervical and salivary gland irradiation that may cause xerostomy. Teeth that can no longer be treated should be extracted with precaution; cavities should be filled; regular application of fluorine is recommended; and any dental prothesis should systematically be checked in order to avoid any irritation of the gums (Carl et al., 1972).

Minor surgical procedures should be kept to a minimum and done aseptically when they are necessary, placing of catheters, etc. Tracheotomized patients should have their canula changed once a day.

When possible, nutritional and metabolic balance should be assured, sometimes at the price of parenteral hyperalimentation, or even better, of gastric catheter. Alcoholics should stop drinking, smokers should no longer smoke; this is desirable both for the immediate and long-term risks of new cancer localizations.

All neoplastic ulcerations should be carefully and regularly disinfected whenever possible, even if there is no major superinfection. This is particularly true for head and neck or female genital cancers.

Most of these measures are included in the reduction of the number of microorganisms, and they can be extended in some cases, as we shall see. We shall now discuss more specific measures: immunoprophylaxis, prophylactic antibiotic therapy, and isolation units.

## Immunoprophylaxis

A variety of vaccines or other immunologic prophylaxis can be proposed and should be discussed. A *priori*, it may seem illogical and ineffective, even dangerous, to try to stimulate immunologic reactions in immunosuppressed patients.

Live or attenuated vaccines should be used only with the greatest caution. We have seen, in fact, that certain agents, known for their low (or even absence of) pathogenicity, cause severe disease in certain compromised patients. A few cases with fatal evolution have been reported consequent to either smallpox vaccination, which produced systemic and lethal vaccina (Hoffbrand, 1964), or to measles vaccination (Mitus *et al.*, 1962). The measles vaccination can also cause giant cell pneumonia (Bodey, 1975). However, we have had sufficient experience with the BCG test, which corresponds to a BCG vaccination, so as not to excessively amplify the risks. As we have stated in Chapter 2, the risks of a localized BCG reaction are very slight (1/5000), even though these tests are usually applied to patients with malignant blood diseases. We have never observed a systemic reaction to BCG. Since this test has been in routine use in our patients (it is considered as an immunologic investigation), we have not observed any cases of tuberculosis in patients followed for nearly 10 years. This experience leads us, perhaps, not to recommend systematic vaccination for all cancer patients, but certainly to recommend it in patients who are exposed to a contagious risk. Moreover, this BCG vaccination and perhaps other vaccinations (?) could delay the progression of malignant lymphomas, as observed by Sokal *et al.* (1974).

With an inactivated vaccine, vaccination is not hazardous and each autumn we advise our patients, who seem particularly susceptible to a severe influenza, to be vaccinated. The only risk is that the vaccination may not work and the patient remains either nonimmunized or insufficiently immunized (but no vaccination is 100% efficacious).

Vaccination studies against *Pseudomonas aeruginosa* have been done in adults and children with cancer. In the adult, an immunization by the seven main immunotypes of lipopolysaccharides which, for example, are active in burn cases, has a moderate but significant efficacy (Young et al., 1973). In the leukemic child, the same type of vaccination initiated in patients in complete remission is accompanied by an increase in antibodies; this increase is observed in most patients but it is transitory and almost only IgM type. This responsive defect is linked to the anti-leukemic maintenance chemotherapy which is continued and in addition, vaccinated children have just as many infections caused by *Pseudomonas* as the control group (Haghbin et al., 1973). In all cases, a severe neutropenia is responsible, for a minimal number of granulocytes are necessary to provide a correct defence against this microorganism (Pennington et al., 1975).

A vaccine agaist *Staphylococcus* may be useful in certain services (Oberling et al., 1975). The frequency of cryptococcosis in patients with Hodgkin's disease in the United States has lead to a proposal for a vaccination against this fungus (Sokal, 1966), but to our knowledge no results have been published.

A vaccine with an attenuated varicella virus has been successfully used in children with cancer (Hattori et al., 1976).

The immunoglobulin supply brings about a more satisfying immunoprophylaxis than vaccination because it does not call upon the failing immunity of the patient. An exogenous supply of gammaglobulins is particularly indicated in patients with type-B lymphoproliferative cancers, such as myelomas and chronic lymphoid leukemias. However, large quantities must be administered in order to be efficacious (0.6–1.8 ml/kg); this seems difficult to renew every 21 days for the rest of the patient's lifetime. A double-blind study concerning intramuscular injection of 20 ml gammaglobulin or a placebo administered every 15 days over a period of a few months did not show any difference in the development of infection in patients with myeloma (Salmon et al., 1967). In addition, current immunoglobulin preparations, which mainly contain IgG, do not seem to have an influence on respiratory or digestive infections (Janeway and Rosen, 1966). Perhaps new immunoglobulin preparations mainly containing IgA could be more effective. Finally, it appears that recipients, after a certain time, may become immunized against these gammaglobulins and thus their effects may be progressively suppressed (Johnson et al., 1972). The recovery of an appropriate rate of autologous immunoglobulins by reduction of neoplastic clones is certainly a preferable measure.

The prophylaxis of herpes zoster and varicella, whose frequency and severity in children with cancer has already been mentioned, by purified gammaglobulins from donors who have a high titer of specific antibodies seems, however, altogether justified in particularly susceptible patients and in epidemic periods. Several controlled studies have demonstrated that nonspecific gammaglobulins have a minor effect, whereas the administration of specific immunoglobulin avoids the appearance of the eruption or significantly diminishes its gravity (Gershon *et al.*, 1974; Geiser *et al.*, 1975; Gaiffe *et al.*, 1976). Specific immunoglobulins are also available for measles (Bodey, 1975) and the number of these products will probably continue to expand over the next few years.

### Prophylactic Antibiotic Therapy

Prophylactic antibiotic therapy can be either systemic or can involve only the digestive tract. It has been particularly studied, accompanied or not by complementary isolation, in the treatment of acute leukemias (Levine *et al.*, 1972).

For many years antibiotics were given prophylactically to all patients who were exposed to developed local or general infection. Generally speaking, in oncology and elsewhere, this treatment has proved to be, at the best, ineffective and, at the worst, harmful by selecting resistant germs which can later cause more severe infections than the infection which would have developed if no treatment had been undertaken (Klastersky, 1971).

Systemic antimicrobial treatment, especially in oncology, does not reduce the frequency of urinary infections in women with genital cancer treated by radium therapy (Wildholm and Mattsson, 1972). In leucopenic patients (between 1000 and 2000/mm$^3$) it was established that intravenous administration of tetracycline was not toxic, but totally useless (Durand *et al.*, 1974). The administration of a broad-spectrum antibiotic in neutropenic and apyretic leukemic patients, who were receiving nondiffusible intestinal antibiotics at the same time, did not avoid or delay the appearance of fever and can favor the development of Gram-negative visceral foci (Dao *et al.*, 1973). In another controlled trial concerning ulcerated cancers of the upper respiratory and digestive tract, the administration of an antibiotic with a more or less broad spectrum was also ineffective in preventing bronchopulmonary complications or general infections (Durand *et al.*, 1975).

The question can then be asked if the best prevention of grave infections is not in restricting systematic antibiotic therapy; certain observations substantiate this position but they have been made in intensive care services and these patients differ from cancer patients (Rapin *et al.*, 1975). However, an interesting controlled study should be mentioned concerning patients operated for cancer of the colon or rectum; 1 g of ampicillin applied on the tissues of the abdominal wall significantly reduced the frequency of postoperative infections without causing secondary adverse effects (particularly on wound healing) (Andersen *et al.*, 1972). These findings confirm those generally obtained with narrow-spectrum antibiotics administered prior to surgery (Campbell, 1965).

Antibiotic therapy may also be administered orally, with drugs that are practically not absorbed, to try to reduce the intestinal flora, which are often the source of endogenous infections (see Chapter 3). Former observations suggested that infectious hazards have thus been reduced in patients with acute lymphoid leukemia (Schwartz *et al.*, 1965). In fact, the majority of these studies involved patients with acute leukemia. In a retrospective study, neomycin B administered orally apparently reduced the frequency of septicemias, but not that of pneumonias (Keating and Penington, 1973). The association of gentamicin, vancomycin, and nystatin accompanied by an alimentation which is either sterile or has a reduced number of microorganisms seemed to reduce general infectious risks (Preisler *et al.*, 1970). However, with the same treatment, another group noted an apparent decrease in bacterial infections, but an increase in fungal infections (Levi *et al.*, 1973). This latter group had difficulty in treating fungal infections with nystatin, but found amphotericin B more efficacious and current publications are in favor of its administration to avoid fungal infections, at least in patients receiving antibiotic therapy for other reasons (Klastersky, 1972).

Whether this reduction of microbial endogenous contamination is efficacious or not, it can have consequences on various digestive metabolisms of the patient, as well as on their coagulation (Dietrich *et al.*, 1973; Yates and Holland, 1973; Cohen *et al.*, 1976). When the patient's digestive tract has been effectively sterilized, special care must be taken during the recovery to assure a recontamination by a benign flora to avoid preferential development of pathogenic microorganisms.

Two controlled studies have demonstrated that reducing the endogenous flora only decreases infections in patients placed in isolation units (Levine *et al.*, 1973; Yates and Holland, 1973). However, other studies demonstrate an efficacious reduction of infections with oral antibiotics, even without isolation units (Klastersky *et al.*, 1974; Schimpff *et al.*, 1975).

However, a less favorable aspect should be emphasized. A retrospective comparison has already indicated that these anti-infectious measures do not modify the rate of leukemic remissions (Bodey *et al.*, 1971). The two controlled studies confirmed that the same rate of remissions was observed in all groups of patients and in addition, their duration was identical (Levine *et al.*, 1973; Yates and Holland, 1973). A more recent publication concerning adults with nonlymphoid acute leukemia and noninfected at the onset indicates that antibiotics administered orally, with or without patient isolation, reduces infectious complications and increases the remission rate by prolonging the median survival of the patients (Schimpff *et al.*, 1975); in this last study it is isolation in a laminar air flow room which seems useless.

These differences can be explained by the variation in patient recruitment (all patients or only uninfected patients), the type of acute leukemia (lymphoid and/or nonlymphoid), the antibiotic therapy administered, the type of isolation, and the type of antileukemic treatment applied. From present studies it does not yet seem possible to make precise conclusions on the efficacy of this antibiotic therapy. In fact it must be considered in close relation to isolation.

### Isolation

Over the last few years the installation of isolation units has developed (Bodey, 1973). The isolation of noninfected patients in special isolation units seems to substantially reduce the frequency of infections in a noncontrolled study (Schneider *et al.*, 1969). Associated with oral antibiotic therapy, this isolation reduced the frequency of infections in patients with a variety of tumors (Levitan and Perry, 1968; Bodey and Rodriguez, 1975). The association of antibiotics seemed useful to Levi *et al.* (1973), but useless to Yates and Holland (1973) in their controlled study. Until now there has been no controlled study which confirms the efficacy of isolation units. The various types of isolation units currently used permit a more or less complete isolation and cause certain difficulties both for the medical staff and the patients (about 1/5 of the patients are immediately excluded for psychologic reasons) and hence these measures still need further research.

### Conclusion

A very limited area of oncology—the acute leukemias, particularly nonlymphoid—has provided important research in order to better control infections in these patients. Three important controlled studies have been published, but their results are not conclusive (Levine *et al.*, 1973; Yates and Holland, 1973; Schimpff *et al.*, 1975). The association of isolation and a reduction of the endogenous flora of the digestive tract by oral antibiotic therapy seems to diminish the risks of superinfection, at least in some cases, but it has not yet been demonstrated that this effect improves the results of antileukemic treatment. These debatable and limited benefits must obviously be considered in relation to their material and personnel inconveniences.

The limited character of present studies should not eliminate this field of research, which remains very interesting. However, more simple measures should be emphasized for the reduction of an endogenous microbial flora prior to placing patients in bone marrow aplasia. Indispensable measures are general hospital hygiene, careful research for a focus with a potential pathogenic microorganism in a leukemic patient at the time of diagnosis, and its sterilization before antileukemic treatment is undertaken. It is also necessary to look for more efficacious and less toxic antileukemic treatments (Yates and Holland, 1973). In addition, the increasing availability of leukocytic concentrates offers a solution of substitution which is more physiologic, and whose efficacy appears more and more evident (Boggs, 1974). The efficacy of prophylactic and isolated leuko cyte transfusion against *E. coli* septicemia has been demonstrated in dogs (Tobias *et al.*, 1976). Studies in this area are now underway in human patients with acute nonlymphoid leukemia. This type of treatment will be discussed in detail in Chapter 10.

CHAPTER 10

# Curative Treatment

The curative treatment of infection, which is favored by impaired host defense mechanisms, often disseminated, and caused by opportunist microorganisms that are often resistant to antibiotic therapy, depends on two types of action: a specific anti-infectious therapy, when one exists, and a substitutive treatment for the inefficacious host defenses.

## ANTI-INFECTIOUS CHEMOTHERAPY

Theoretically, anti-infectious chemotherapy presupposes that the etiologic agent is known, for treatment varies depending on the microorganism; however, as we have previously stated, this is not always possible and an empiric treatment must often be undertaken. Moreover, the rapid evolution of some infections necessitates an immediate anti-infectious chemotherapy. Clinically, when a cancer patient has fever, especially if he is granulopenic (Schimpff *et al.*, 1971; Tattersall *et al.*, 1972; Symposium, 1973; Klastersky *et al.*, 1975; Aubertin, *et al.*, 1977), it can be assumed that a microorganism is responsible (Table XXXIV).

### Treatment of Identified Infections

The choice and the means of therapy depend on the site of the infection and the etiologic agent. Its ways and means have been partly discussed in Chapters 5–8. Here we shall recall the general rules of identification and administration of it.

**Bacterial Infections.** These mainly depend on antibiotic therapy. However, an antibiotic's eventual adverse effects in cancer patients should be kept in mind. We have already stressed the possible role played by broad-spectrum antibiotics in the development of fungal infections and/ or infections caused by muliresistant Gram-negative bacteria. When the microorganism responsible for the infection has been identified, it is then tested for *in vitro* sensitivity and an appropriate antibiotic therapy is chosen.

140

TABLE XXXIV. Management of Febrile Cancer Patients

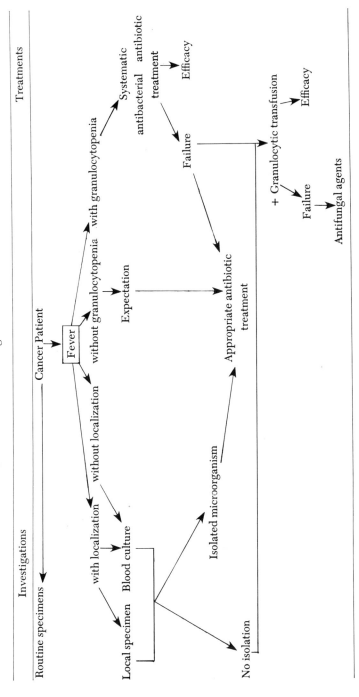

*Principles.* The antibiotic or antibiotics chosen should be bactericidal. Bacteriostatic antibiotics generally cannot eradicate infection when host defenses are impaired. Thus beta-lactamines (penicillins, cephalosporins), aminosides, polypeptides (colistine, polymyxine B), and rifampycin represent the best group of antibiotics. Each group of antibiotics has preferential indications. In the study of Klastersky (1971) (Fig. 15), which dealt with the sensitivity of microorganisms isolated from cancer patients, gentamicin and polymyxin are the most active on *Escherichia coli* and *Klebsiella*, while gentamicin, cephalothin, and·carbenicillin are the best antibiotics against *Proteus mirabilis,* and carbenicillin, polymyxine, and gentamicin are active on a little more than half of the *Pseudomonas.* Other antibiotics, used since 1971, are also useful against Gram-negative bacilli. Amikacin, an aminoside derived from kanamycin, has an activity spectrum similar to that of gentamicin but is presently efficacious against the majority of bacilli resistant to gentamicin (Meyer *et al.,* 1975; Tally *et al.,* 1975; Pollak *et al.,* 1977). Ticarcillin, a beta-lactamine close to carbenicillin, has the same efficacy as carbenicillin but with 30–50% lower dosages; this fact may reduce the side effects (eosinophilia, hypokalemia, coagulation disorders) (Ervin and Bullock, 1976;

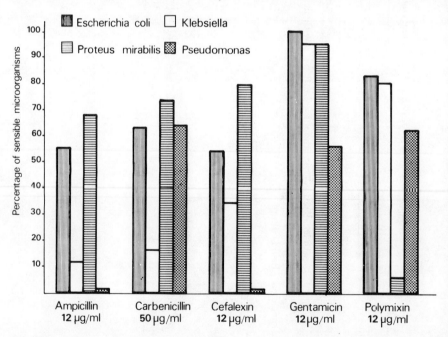

**Fig. 15.** Sensitivity of main Gram-negative bacilli to some antibiotics (from Klastersky, 1971).

Parry and Neu, 1976). In another study, Klastersky *et al.* (1973) demonstrated the frequency of cross-resistances between different aminoglycosides such as gentamicin, tobramycin, sisomycin, and the more frequent activity of gentamicin on *E. coli*, tobramycin on *Pseudomonas*, and sisomycin on *E. coli, Klebsiella, Proteus*, and *Staphylococcus*. However, even bactericidal antibiotics have a reduced efficacy in patients with severe granulocytopenia (Middleman *et al.*, 1972; Bodey and Rodriguez, 1973; Klastersky *et al.*, 1975). Bactericidal action is obtained only with sufficient concentration, larger than bacteriostatic concentrations. In severe infections it is often useful to determine the minimal bactericidal concentration of an antibiotic on the isolated microorganism, so that the prescribed dose is appropriate. The efficacy of the treatment is all the more probable as the minimal inhibitory concentration (or even better the minimal bactericidal concentration) of the antibiotic on the bacteria is low (Tillotson and Finland, 1969).

Bactericidal action can be obtained by the association of two antibiotics if they are synergistic (Bastin *et al.*, 1971; Klastersky, 1972). Theoretically there is a strong synergy between the beta-lactamines and the aminosides (Jawetz, 1968). In addition, the beta-lactamines which are resistant to penicillinase, have an affinity for certain forms of beta-lactamases secreted by the Gram-negative bacteria and can neutralize them (Sabath and Abraham, 1964). Therefore the cephalosporins may be associated with a penicillin sensitive to penicillinase, such as ampicillin, carbenicillin, or ticarcilline thus liberated from the action of the penicillinase (Klastersky, 1973; Schimpff *et al.*, 1976).

There may be a difference between the *in vitro* and *in vivo* activity of an antibiotic. Several recent studies indicate results obtained with certain antibiotic associations. Table XXXV shows some disagreement on the efficacy of an antibiotic alone or in association in the same family of microorganisms. On *Pseudomonas*, carbenicillin used alone acts less well than when it is associated with another antibiotic; except for the cephalothin–gentamicin combination which is not very efficacious, a variety of combinations give similar results.

For *Proteus*, the carbenicillin–cephalothin and cephalothin–gentamicin combinations are less active than carbenicillin–gentamicin or carbenicillin–cephalothin–gentamicin combinations (Klastersky *et al.*, 1974).

For *E. coli* the carbenicillin–cephalothin, ampicillin–gentamicin, and carbenicillin–cephalothin–gentamicin combinations give results similar to those of gentamicin used alone.

For the group of microorganisms including *Klebsiella–Enterobacter–Serratia*, only *Klebsiella* are sensitive to cephalothin which may be combined with gentamicin, carbenicillin, or both.

TABLE XXXV. Efficacy of Main Antibiotics on Diverse Microorganisms

| Antibiotics | Pseudomonas | Proteus | E. coli | Klebsiella Enterobacter Serratia | Other Gram-Negative Agents | Gram-Positive Microorganisms | All Microorganisms | References |
|---|---|---|---|---|---|---|---|---|
| Gentamicin | 45% | 100% | 75% | 45–60% | 67% | 50% | | Bodey et al. (1972) |
| Carbenicillin | 6/12 | 3/5 | 2/5 | | | | 50% | Klastersky et al. (1973) |
| | 12/13 | 3/6 | 0 | | 0/7 | | 57% | Bloomfield and Kennedy (1974) |
| Carbenicillin + gentamicin | 3/3 | 2/2 | 1/4 | 1/1 | 6/12 | | 57% | Rodriguez et al. (1969) |
| | 17/21 | | 5/7 | | 8/20 | | 60% | Schimpff et al. (1971) |
| | 9/10 | | 0/3 | 4/10 | 1/1 | 3/4 | 82% | Klastersky et al. (1973) |
| Carbenicillin + kanamycin | 8/9 | 4/5 | 2/3 | 2/5 | | 3/4 | 66% | Middleman et al. (1972) |
| Carbenicillin + cephalothin | 6/7 | 5/8 | 8/10 | 9/10 | 4/5 | | 70% | Middleman et al. (1972) |
| Cephalothin + gentamicin | 10/12 | 2/6 | 4/6 | 8/9 | | | 80% | Klastersky et al. (1974) |
| Ampicillin + gentamicin | 2/5 | 3/7 | 8/12 | 1/12 | | | 61% | Klastersky et al. (1971) |
| Cephalothin + tobramycin | 4/6 | | 7/13 | 4/11 | 3/6 | 4/4 | 60% | Klastersky et al. (1971) |
| Ticarcillin + tobramycin | 2/8 | | 9/13 | 2/7 | 1/3 | 5/11 | 48% | Klastersky et al. (1975) |
| Ticarcillin + cephalothin | 8/10 | | 10/14 | 2/5 | 4/6 | 6/9 | 57% | |
| Ticarcillin + gentamicin | 3/5 | | 2/3 | 5/11 | | 5/6 | 63% | |
| Ticarcillin + cephalothin | 1/3 | | 1/4 | 1/4 | | 8/8 | 63% | |
| | 3/4 | | | | | | 64% | Schimpff et al. (1976) |
| Carbenicillin + cephalothin + gentamicin | 5/6 | | 9/11 | 15/17 | | 4/4 | 86% | Bloomfield and Kennedy (1974) |
| | 5/8 | 10/12 | 8/10 | 5/18 | | | 76% | Klastersky et al. (1974) |

The cephalo–tobramycin, ticarcillin–gentamicin, ticarcillin–tobramycin, and ticarcillin–cephalothin combinations studied by Klastersky et al., (1975) and Schimpff et al., (1976) in a variety of infections, mainly those caused by Gram-negative bacilli, did not give better results.

The efficacy of combined sulfamethoxazole–trimethoprim has recently been pointed out (Grose et al., 1977). These drugs are given orally, every 8 hr, at daily doses of 800 mg sulfamethoxazole and 160 mg trimethoprim; in 36 patients with pneumonia or septicemia resistant to the carbenicillin–aminoglycoside combination this treatment induced recovery in 54% of the cases. For this combination no correlation seems to exist between minimum inhibitory concentration and clinical response.

The efficacy of the antibiotic treatment is influenced by the diffusion of the antibiotic at the site of infection. This aspect is often overlooked in the choice of an antibiotic. Moreover, the diffusion of substances varies; certain antibiotics cannot diffuse in the meninges.

The adverse effects of some antibiotic treatments should not be overlooked. High doses of beta-lactamines and aminosides can provoke renal insufficiency, phlebitis, hypokaliemia, erythema, hemorrhages, deafness, vertigo, eosinophilia, and superinfections in 2–20% of the cases (Klastersky et al., 1975; Table XXXVI). The renal toxicity of the association cephalothin–gentamicin is higher when there is another discrete impairment of renal functions, for example, in case of hemorrhage or owing to the infection itself (Plager, 1976). However, it can be decreased by a high daily urine output.

*Indications.* Certain local bacterial infections only need localized treatment. These are superficial cutaneous infections and sometimes even superficial infections of the upper respiratory tract and digestive cancers. Local antiseptics may be sufficient.

Pulmonary infection is difficult to identify (see Chapter 5). It is generally treated by broad-spectrum antibiotic treatments; their compared effects are shown in Table XXXVII from some recent publications. For Klastersky et al. (1973), carbenicillin–gentamicin is more efficacious than carbenicillin or gentamicin used alone; but, these results vary from one study to another. Israel (1972) notes favorable results with just cotrimoxazole in 40 out of 50 lung cancers complicated by respiratory infections. Local use of antibiotics may be useful. Among 15 cancer patients with tracheotomy, 7 were treated with gentamicin endotracheally for bronchial infection and all 7 recovered; 8 received the same drug but by intramuscular injection and only 2 recovered (Klastersky et al., 1972).

Urinary infections are certainly much easier to treat. The responsible

TABLE XXXVI. Side Effects of Antibiotics in Cancer Patients

| Antibiotics | Renal Failure[a] | Phlebitis | Hypokalemia | Erythema | Hemorrhages | Super-infection | References |
|---|---|---|---|---|---|---|---|
| Carbenicillin + cephalothin | 8 | | | | | | |
| Carbenicillin + kanamycin | 12 | | | | | | Middleman et al. (1972) |
| Cephalothin + tobramycin | 21 | 22 | 2 | 6,5 | | 16 | |
| Ticarcillin + tobramycin | 6 | 26 | 16 | 0 | 0 | 12 | Klastersky et al. (1975) |
| Ticarcillin + cephalothin | 2 | 27 | 30 | 4 | 4 | 13 | |
| Cephalothin + carbenicillin + gentamicin | 25 | | 60 | 10 | 4 | | Bloomfield and Kennedy (1974) |

[a] Figures are percentage.

TABLE XXXVII.  Efficacy of Antibiotic Regimens on Various Types of Infections

| Antibiotics | Septicemias | Respiratory Infections | Urinary Infections | Cellulitis | All Infections | References |
|---|---|---|---|---|---|---|
| Gentamicin | 41% | 47% | 82% | | | Bodey et al. (1972) |
| | 45% | | | | | Bodey et al. (1972) |
| | 1/3 | 7/12 | 3/4 | | 58% | Klastersky et al. (1973) |
| Carbenicillin | 15/19 | 2/3 | 6/7 | 4/7 | 75% | Bodey et al. (1969) |
| | 48/59 | 9/14 | | | 78% | Bodey et al. (1971) |
| | 2/4 | 4/9 | 2/4 | | 47% | Klatersky et al. (1973) |
| Ticarcillin | 92% | | | | | Bodey et al. (1971) |
| Carbenicillin+gentamicin | 47% | | | | 47% | Rodriguez et al. (1969) |
| | 11/13 | | | | 84% | Schimpff et al. (1971) |
| | 4/5 | 8/10 | 1/2 | | 76% | Klatersky et al. (1973) |
| Carbenicillin+kanamycin | 8/15 | 13/25 | 1/1 | | 53% | Middleman et al. (1972) |
| Carbenicillin+cephalothin | 6/10 | 12/23 | 4/4 | | 59% | Middleman et al. (1972) |
| | 16/20 | 6/9 | 2/2 | | 77% | Klatersky et al. (1974) |
| Cephalothin+tobramycin | 11/9 | 2/13 | 5/6 | 1/4 | 53% | Klatersky et al. (1975) |
| Ticarcillin+tobramycin | 7/15 | 9/14 | 4/6 | 2/3 | 53% | |
| Ticarcillin+cephalothin | 6/11 | 6/11 | 3/4 | 3/6 | 61% | |
| Carbenicillin+cephalothin +gentamicin | 15/9 | 7/13 | 2/2 | | 71% | Klatersky et al. (1974) |

microorganisms are easily identified; the beta-lactamines and aminosides give high urinary concentrations. It is not necessary to combine two antibiotics.

Septicemias are a serious problem. Even though they are bacteriologically confirmed and appropriately treated they do not always respond favorably for several reasons: impaired host immunity, virulence of the microorganism, and sometimes superinfection, particularly fungal. The efficacy of the treatment varies between 40 and 90% according to the particular study; bactericidal associations are more active than single antibiotic treatment (Table XXXV).

**Fungal Infections.** Therapy is readily simple in cutaneous or superficial mucous membrane candidiasis: application of skin dyes and washing of the mucous membranes with nystatin or amphotericin B.

Esophageal candidiasis is more difficult to treat. Nystatin or amphotericin B administered orally are sometimes insufficient for, unlike the fungus, these antibiotics do not penetrate in depth into mucous membranes. On the contrary, flucytosine diffuses well and can be used in these *Candida* infections.

Deep visceral infections, pulmonary or meningeal, as well as fungal septicemias still depend on antibiotics with limited diffusibility: ampothericin B, flucytosine, and clotrimazole.

We have already discussed the modes of treatment for these infections (see Chapter 7), and have also emphasized the difficulties in the treatment of aspergillosis in comparison with candidiasis, and of phycomycosis in comparison with the aforementioned. In the latter, 9–12 ml of a saturated solution of potassium iodine in 24 hr gives some aid as amphothericin B and flucytosine are not very efficacious (Bennett, 1974). We shall point out the utility of nystatin or amphotericin in aerosols for pulmonary candidiasis or aspergillosis (Burke and Coltman, 1971). We have also stressed intrathecal treatment by amphotericin in cryptococcosis (Diamond and Bennett, 1974).

**Viral Infections.** Actually there are no current medicines which are efficacious in the treatment of hepatitis and cytomegalic inclusions disease.

In herpes virus infections and in particular herpes zoster and varicella, the real efficacy of cytarabine or parental administration of idoxuridine has not yet been universally established (see Chapter 6). The unfavorable evolution of these infections in immunodepressed patients, and particularly in leukemias, authorizes the use of cytotoxic drugs. But if certain studies show a shortening in the duration of evolution, even an improvement in overall prognosis, others conclude the inefficacy of these treatments in randomized studies, and even to the aggravation of the immunosuppression.

Adenine–arabinoside is less toxic and seems more efficacious according to the experience of Ch'ien *et al.* (1976). In a randomized trial, adenine–arabinoside shortens the duration of herpes zoster in young patients with malignant lymphoma if it is administered early (Whitley *et al.*, 1976). Moreover, it also seems to affect cytomegalovirosis, herpetic encephalitis, and generalized herpes (Aronson *et al.*, 1976).

**Parasitic Infections.** Their therapy has been discussed in Chapter 7. The indications depend on the diagnosis, and are particularly difficult for infections caused by *Pneumocystis*.

## Therapy in Nonidentified Infections

Any fever in patients with immune deficiency, and particularly in patients with leukemia and granulocytopenia, is suspected of having an infectious origin. *A priori* the association of fever with signs of localization such as a clinical and/or x-ray confirmed pulmonary pathology substantiate this hypothesis, even though dissemination of a cancer can provoke similar reactions.

It is possible to wait for bacteriologic, mycotic, virologic, or parasitologic confirmation, but the eventuality of severe complications, such as infectious shock in septicemias caused by Gram-negative bacilli, makes this waiting dangerous. In addition we have already mentioned the delays of diagnosis in the cases of systemic or visceral fungal disease or in pneumocystosis. Thus a treatment may be undertaken based on simple clinical considerations and corrected after return of further results obtained by biologic investigations which give etiologic answers (Table XXXIV).

In such circumstances a broad-spectrum antibiotic treatment is first indicated. A number of associations have been tried: cephalosporin–aminoglycoside, carbenicillin–aminoglycoside, ticarcillin–aminoglycoside, carbenicillin or ticarcillin and cephalosporin at high doses (200 mg/kg per day of cephalothin, 500 mg/kg per day of carbenicillin, 4–5 mg/kg per day of gentamicin or tobramycin). More complex combinations have been used such as cephalosporin–carbenicillin–aminoglycoside or even combinations with five antibiotics. Results obtained with these treatments depend on the type of infections observed in each hospital. In clinical practice bacterial infections in cancer patients, mainly in granulopenic patients, are due to microorganisms of their endogenous environment (Schimpff *et al.*, 1972). Hence, before identifying the etiologic agent in a febrile cancer patient, antibiotic treatment should not be given arbitrarily but should be adapted to the microbial ecology of the hospital and to the microorganisms isolated by previous systematic cultures from nose, skin, throat, stool and urine of the patient (Nauta and Van Furth, 1975; Aubertin *et al.*, 1977). It is often very useful to associate a beta-lacta-mine and an aminoside because of their usual syngeristic action.

The aforementioned treatment is ineffective in nonbacterial infections. It seems logical to continue a treatment 3 or 4 days, but, after this period if there is no clinical improvement or if the patient's status is aggravated, antibiotic therapy should be replaced by an antifungal treatment com-bining intravenous amphotericin B and flucytosine given either orally or intravenously.

## NONSPECIFIC TREATMENT

The aim of nonspecific treatment is to complete anti-infectious chemo-therapy by acting directly on the circumstances which favor the infection.

### General Measures

It is not necessary to insist on surgical evacuation of a suppuration or the cleaning of an abscess which has spontaneously fistulized, such as perianal abscesses in granulopenic patients. The removal of an obstacle which is the source of a purulent retention, such as those observed in ureteral or bronchial obstructions, is also useful. The obstacle may be eliminated either by surgery or by localized irradiation. Finally, simple removal of a venous or urinary catheter is sufficient in some cases to eliminate the infection, with or without antibiotics.

More important, but also more debatable, are treatments which aim to restore host defenses, either by granulocytic transfusions or by immunoglobulins (Schwarzenberg *et al.*, 1966).

### Blood Fractions

**Leukocytes.** Initially prepared by simple sedimentation from blood of patients with chronic myeloid leukemia in the hyperleukocytic stage, white cell transfusions have profited, in recent years, from immunologic and technical progress. Hence it is now possible to assure a better com-patibility between the leukocytes of the donor and the receiver and to choose a donor from which leukocytic concentration may be prepared by either centrifugation, continuous or discontinuous flow, or by filtration, according to the type of material used (Goldman and Lowenthal, 1975).

The effectiveness of this ample supply of leukocytes has been proved in animals (Epstein *et al.*, 1969). The combination gentamicin and granulocyte transfusions is more efficacious than either the gentamicin–carbenicillin or the carbenicillin–leucocytes combination, or each antibiotic alone, or granulocyte transfusions alone (Dale *et al.*, 1976).

In man, the viability of transfused leukocytes has been demonstrated as well as the increase in the number of circulating leukocytes in the recipients (Boggs, 1974). However, the exact efficacy of these transfusions and their indications in the treatment of infections in granulopenic patients still need further experimentation.

These transfusions have been especially applied to patients with acute leukemia. We have seen that the bactericidal action of certain antibiotic loses a lot of its efficacy when the number of granulocytes falls below 500/mm$^3$ (Bodey and Rodriguez, 1973); in addition, present day isolation units for granulopenic patients are not always completely efficacious (see Chapter 9). Hence, it seems logical that a patient in aplasia should receive viable granulocytes possessing all their enzymatic properties, thus aiding in the antibacterial defense of the host.

Schwarzenberg *et al.* (1966) obtained 12 good clinical results in the treatment of 23 septicemias by transfusions of white blood cells from chronic myeloid leukemic patients. Bussel *et al.* (1971) have transfused 570 leukocytic concentrates to 289 patients during 341 episodes of leukopenia: the mean number of white cells transfused was 10$^{11}$/m$^2$: 67% of thermic defervescences were observed, while in 68% of the patients the increase in the number of leukocytes was more than 2000. The best results were obtained in children with acute lymphoid leukemia.

Graw *et al.* (1972) observed that hardly one-third (11/37) of the septicemias treated by antibiotics alone were cured, while nearly half (18/39) recovered when the antibiotic therapy was associated with leukocytic transfusions. The difference is not significant; the efficacy of the leukocytes is higher when the patients have received numerous transfusions very early at the beginning of the infection.

Lowenthal *et al.* (1975) collected 137 leukocytic concentrates from normal donors, and 78 from patients with chronic myeloid leukemia. Forty-one patients received these concentrates during 89 aplastic episodes with probable or certain infection which had resisted antibiotic therapy. A thermic defervescence was noted in 67% of the cases if two units or more were transfused, and only 24% with a single unit. There is a positive correlation between the increase in the number of neutrophils in the receiver and the thermic defervescene; fever diminishes more rapidly in patients with less than 1000 granulocytes before the transfusion.

Vallejos *et al.* (1975) treated 179 febrile episodes in 128 leukopenic patients; 454 leukocytic transfusions were prepared by centrifugation from patients with chronic myeloid leukemia. All transfusions were administered 1 hr after collection. On the average, $1.3 \times 10^{11}$ granulo-cytes were transfused two times for each infectious episode. The authors observed, on the whole, 49% favorable responses, with apyrexy during 48 hr and clinical and radiologic improvement of infectious symptoms. The median survival of these patients is 21.5 weeks against 2.5 for non-responding patients. The percentage of success is 36% for septicemias with deep infectious foci and 76% for subcutaneous infections. The vari-ations of responses according to the microorganisms responsible for the infection are minimal, but the association of several microorganisms seems to diminish the percentage of good results. Infections caused by *Candida* seem just as sensitive as bacterial infections. Patients over 50 years of age respond less favorably. The percent of leukocytic increase is, in 87% of the cases, less than 20% of the initial number; only 5% of the transfusions provoked a leukocytic increase of more than 40%.

Schiffer *et al.* (1975) transfused 131 leukocytic units in 21 leukopenic patients. Approximately $2.8 \times 10^{11}$ granulocytes were collected by filtra-tion for each transfusion. The number of granulocytes increases on the average of $225/mm^3$ in the blood of the receiver. Three patients recov-ered from their infection, nine survived with their infection stabilized, while eight others died of infectious complications. The authors have some doubts as to the efficacy of these transfusions and outline the difficulties of evaluating this therapy.

However, Higby *et al.* (1975) performed a randomized study on the efficacy of lekocytic transfusion obtained by filtration in leukopenic patients with less than 500 granulocytes/$mm^3$ blood presenting a patent infection after 48 hr of antibiotic treatment. Four transfusions of $2$–$5 \times 10^{11}$ granulocytes were administered in 4 days. Among the 19 nontranfused control patients, 5 were still alive on the 20th day, whereas among the 17 transfused patients, only 2 patients had succumbed by the 20th day; all survivors were apyretic. Age, type of infection, previous treatments, and the nature of the underlying malignancy do not explain these differences. Hence, the authors consider that the granulocytes obtained by filtration are efficacious in overcoming infections in leuko-penic patients.

On the whole, the results of leukocytic transfusions seem satisfying but, owing to the lack of common evaluation criteria concerning the efficacy of these transfusions, and lack of a control group receiving only antibiotic therapy, these results are not yet conclusive as to the real utility of these transfusions.

Two recent randomized trials afford some interesting data. Thirty Gram-negative septicemias in 27 cancer patients with bone marrow aplasia were included in the first trial (Herzig *et al.*, 1977); 12 out of

16 patients receiving daily leukocyte transfusions survived while 9 out of 14 patients receiving only antibiotics died. The most important prognosis factor is the spontaneous leukocyte recovery: leukocyte transfusions are useless in patients recovering a normal leukocyte production but are useful for patients remaining in aplasia. In a second trial, 19 leukemic patients with bone marrow aplasia and fever were treated by antibiotics alone and 12 patients received antibiotic treatment associated with daily leukocyte transfusions (Alavi *et al.*, 1977): only 20% of the patients receiving only antibiotic treatment were alive by the 21st day versus 75% of the patients receiving $3.2 \times 10^{10}$ granulocytes every day. The usefulness of leukocytes is more marked in patients with long-lasting aplasia and bacteriologically proven infection than in patients with fever of unknown origin and recovering normal bone marrow production before the 21st day.

At the same time, Boggs (1977) points out that the benefit of these transfusions is still disputable, and is without significant effect on patient survival rate. Moreover, there are difficulties in collecting leukocytes, thus the cost/benefit ratio does not seem worthwhile.

Thus it would be very important to determine exactly what types of patient benefit from these leukocyte transfusions and what types of patients do not. Besides it would be useful to improve and to simplify the technique of leukopheresis. This is the objective of the studies which are now underway.

**Gammaglobulins.** When patients with a definite hypogammaglobulinemia develop infections it seems logical to give them immunoglobulins (Ig) and generally a dose of 1–2 ml/kg of weight is advised. Such a treatment would be paradoxically useful for infections which complicate acute leukemias, even if there is no confirmed deficiency in serum immunoglobulins. However, the usual preparations contain practically only IgG and low percentages of IgA, which explain their very debatable efficacy in mucous membrane infections of the digestive and respiratory tract. In addition, the possibility of local intramuscular or general intolerance after intravenous injection cannot be overlooked; finally, antibodies may develop after repeated injections and may reduce the therapeutic efficacy, but their real importance is debatable (Johnson *et al.*, 1972).

These inconveniences and a limited efficacy explain the reticence expressed on this treatment and justify research attempts toward the preparation of specific immunoglobulins which may be administered prophylactically (see Chapter 9) but may also be effective in attenuating an already established infection.

# CHAPTER 11

# Evolution and Prognosis

In a cancer patient an infection often constitutes an unfavorable factor either because it is a sign of an advanced stage of the cancer or because the infection itself is a serious menace.

It is altogether exceptional that the *development of an infection is accompanied by an improvement in the cancer.* A few isolated cases have been published and several observations of spontaneous regression coincide with a severe infection (Everson and Cole, 1966). Attempts have been made to link these facts to immunologic stimulation afforded by the infection. However, "treatment" studies of Hodgkin's disease, by transmission of viral hepatitis, based on such observations, were rapidly discontinued (Hoster *et al.*, 1949). Encouraging results obtained with an attenuated mumps virus need to be confirmed (Asada, 1974). There are a number of reports dealing with lung cancer and post-operative infections. In some series, patients who develop empyema after surgical resection of pulmonary tumor seem to survive longer than patients without infectious complication (Takita, 1970; Ruckdeschel *et al.*, 1972). For example, the 5-year survival rate for patients with empyema is 50% versus 18% in control noninfected patients (Ruckde-schel *et al.*, 1972). However, in other series, the survival is lower in patients with postoperative empyema in comparison with patients with-out infection (Cady and Clifton, 1967; Lawton and Keehn, 1972). Never-theless, these data stimulated McKneally *et al.* (1976) to carry out a randomized trial to study the effects of intrapleural BCG after surgery for lung cancer: BCG significantly improved the survival of patients with a limited tumor, while it did not seem to be beneficial in patients with more advanced diseases. Perhaps intratumoral injection of BCG should be included here also (Sparks *et al.*, 1973) or even every kind of "immunotherapy" using living microorganisms.

Often infection develops in cancer patients as it does in healthy subjects, has a usual evolution, and heals without particular compli-cations. Patients in complete remission and without maintenance treat-ment are evidently susceptible to any passing infection, as is the general population. Even if the cancer is evolving or the patient is in treatment, the infection may have a simple evolution. Thus the appearance of cytomegalic inclusion disease in leukemic patients does not seem to modify the prognosis (Sutton *et al.*, 1971; Bussel *et al.*, 1975); banal herpes zoster infection in any cancer patient also seems to be without significance.

However, in many cases, especially when the evolution of the cancer cannot be controlled, the infection is particularly severe and can cause the death of the patient. This work is concerned with all of these infections because they are particular to cancer patients and their severity poses special clinical and therapeutic problems.

## INTERLOCKING PATHOLOGY

Infections in cancer patients may correspond to several types of "pathologic mesh" (Hoerni, 1972) where one illness predisposes to a second disease or even to a third one (Table XXXVIII). We shall discuss the main mechanisms.

The first one originates from cancer which predisposes to an infection by multiple ways (see Chapter 3). Its influence may be direct when it creates a break in a primary barrier or by mechanical disturbances of drainage or general immune deficiency. It can be indirect by the intermediary, i.e., the treatment necessitated by the cancer. This is the reason why the severest infections are observed during the severest cancers. This severity is due to either the type of cancer or its evolutive stage, not only because these cancers cause important local or general disturbances, but also because they necessitate particularly toxic treatments which may aggravate (at least temporarily) the fragility of the patient, who is especially vulnerable toward infectious agents. An evolutive

TABLE XXXVIII. Schematic Representation of an Interlocking Pathology Leading from Cancer to Infections

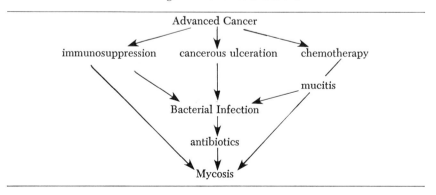

parallel is observed in Hodgkin's disease: the initial insufficiency of cell-mediated immune response predisposes mainly for viral infections, particularly to herpes zoster with benign evolution; later, if the lymphoma has not been controlled and evolves with aggravation of the general status of the patient, a decrease of humoral defenses appears, and at this stage, complicated viral, bacterial, and fungal infections are found (Hoerni *et al.*, 1971). In a number of patients one cancer predisposes to many infections (Table XXXIX).

There are also several types of interlocking factors where the infection predisposes to infection; this is true for pathology on the whole, but particularly in compromised patients. The mechanism which is probably the most common, or at least the best understood, involves the influence of antibiotics. Their application, if it is prolonged, even when fully

TABLE XXXIX.  Example of Sequential Infections in a Cancer Patient

Miss X (FB 72 0917), 17 years old

Hodgkin's disease, clinical stage IIB (mediastinal + supraclavicular lymphadenopathy), scleronodular type, treated by chemotherapy + radiotherapy, between May 15, 1972 and June 7, 1972. The patient is still in complete remission in July 1976.

Infections
  (1) Rubella:
        Clinical: June 1972 skin rash
        Serology (hemagglutination inhibition test)

| | |
|---|---|
| July 6, 1972 | 1/20,480 |
| October 13, 1972 | 1/640 |
| November 20, 1972 | 1/640 |

  (2) Herpes zoster:
        December 1972, abdominocrural localization, benign evolution.
  (3) Toxoplasmosis:
        Ocular localization. First symptoms in September 1973.
        Dye test:

| | |
|---|---|
| May 18, 1972 | 50 International Units |
| April 4, 1973 | 2,000 I.U. |
| December 10, 1973 | 3,600 I.U. |
| May 27, 1974 | 2,900 I.U. |

Comments
  (1) Rubella resulted in a monoclonal gammapathy and other biologic disturbances like increase of erythrocyte sedimentation rate which, for a few months, prevented the affirmation of complete remission of Hodgkin's disease after radiotherapy.
  (2) Ocular toxoplasmosis was first considered as possible tumor.

justified, causes modifications in the patient's microbial flora and selects microorganisms which are resistant and generally more virulent. This phenomenon is observed for certain bacterial infections and is above all the source of fungal infections (see Chapter 7). However, this treatment is not an indispensable step in order to pass from one infection to another one; it is a well-known fact that viruses create conditions favorable to bacterial infections and this seems particularly true in cancer patients (Bodey, 1975). Herpetic lesions of the respiratory and digestive tracts may become superinfected with *Straphylococcus*, Gram-negative bacilli, or *Candida*. Viral pneumonias also create local favorable conditions for the development of a secondary bacterial or fungal infection. Moreover, this microbial relay often constitutes a main factor in the gravity of viral infections which would otherwise be banal. In a large series of pneumocystosis, one third of the patients had a second associated infection which was bacterial, viral, or fungal, localized or more often disseminated (Walzer *et al.*, 1974). These examples can be easily multiplied by current observations.

In many cases these interlocking factors provoke the patient's death.

## LETHAL INFECTIONS

It is difficult to give a general evaluation of the severity of infections in cancer patients. In a service of infectious diseases, one out of ten infections is severe (Lacut *et al.*, 1974); in a service of medical oncology, for 176 affirmed infections, only one was considered as responsible for the death of the patient (Durand *et al.*, 1974); this divergence can be explained by different recruitment conditions.

However, these infections play an important role among the causes of death in cancer patients.

Two recent papers coming from the Jules-Bordet Institute (Klastersky *et al.*, 1972) and Roswell Park Institute (Ambrus *et al.*, 1975), involving patients necropsied in 1970–1971, give comparable figures for two series concerning, respectively, 157 and 507 patients. Isolated or associated with another cause, infections contribute to the death of the patient in nearly half of the cases (47 and 49%, respectively); alone, they are directly responsible for 32 and 36% of the deaths. Lethal infections are generally caused by Gram-negative bacilli (Table XL). Infection constitutes the only causes of death in 16% of lung cancers, 24% in breast tumors, 25% in malignant lymphomas, and more than half of the genitourinary cancers (53%), respiratory and digestive cancers (54%), and acute leukemias (56%).

In a larger series of 816 cancer patients at the M.D. Anderson Hos-

TABLE XL.   Infections Responsible for Death, Alone or Along with
another Cause in Unselected Cancer Patients[a]

| Microorganism | Type of Infections | | | | | |
|---|---|---|---|---|---|---|
| | Septi-cemia | Pulmonary Infection | Urinary Infection | Wound Infection | Peritonitis | Total |
| *Pneumococcus* | | 1 | | | | 1 |
| *Staphylococcus* | 2 | 6 | | | 2 | 10 |
| *Klebsiella* | 8 | 13 | 1 | 1 | 1 | 24 |
| *Pseudomonas* . | 1 | 5 | 1 | 1 | | 8 |
| *E. coli* | 7 | 3 | 1 | | 3 | 14 |
| *Proteus* | 1 | 3 | 2 | 4 | 4 | 14 |
| Mycobacteria | | 1 | | | | 1 |
| Virus | 1 | 1 | | 1 | | 3 |
| Fungus | 1 | 3 | | | | 4 |

[a] From Klastersky *et al.* (1972); 1970–1971; Institut Jules-Bordet, Brussels, Belgium.

pital necropsied in 1968–1970, dealing only with solid tumors, infection was considered as the main cause of death in 47% (380) of the patients (Inagaki *et al.*, 1974). Half of the cases (192) were peneumonias which developed especially in patients with lung or upper digestive–respiratory tract cancers; almost as often (147), it was a septicemia, particularly frequent in urogenital cancers—mainly gynecologic—or gastrointestinal cancers. Cases of peritonitis and other varied infections were rare. Fatal infection was favored by a necropsing or ulcerated tumor or by compressing physiologic pathways in two-thirds of the patients, by a neutropenia in 14%, and more rarely by a postradiotherapy or postsurgery complication.

In comparison with solid tumors, acute leukemias are more likely to develop fatal infections; they are considered responsible for 70% of deaths by Hersh *et al.* (1965). In a series of 199 necropsied leukemic children, infection constituted the main cause of death in 89 cases and an ancillary cause in 66 others and was thus responsible in various degrees for the death of more than three-quarters of the patients (Hughes, 1971). As in other series, Gram-negative bacilli were mainly responsible for the lethal infections.

In considering only chronic myeloid leukemia, it can be noted that infection was responsible for death twice as often in patients who presented an acute transformation (34%) than in those whose disease remained in a chronic phase (17%) (Monfardini *et al.*, 1973).

Thus infections as causes of death are placed before hemorrhagic accidents and thromboembolisms and are far ahead of cancer itself (which constitutes a direct cause of death only for breast and lung cancers), while common cachexia is responsible for only 1% of the death in patients. However, it should be recognized that very often patients who died with an infection were also patients with very advanced cancers [90% of them in the series of Klastersky *et al.*, (1972)] and it would appear more exact to link the severe infection to the terminal stage of the cancer than to link the death to the infection. However, a better infectious control could delay the fatal issue, and, consequently, deserves much more attention. It is the case, in particular, of some very advanced cancers which could be controlled with treatment whose activity manifests only after a few days or a few weeks provided that an early death caused by infection does not supervene before.

## PROGNOSIS OF INFECTED CANCER PATIENTS

Because the cancer is the source, either directly or indirectly, of infection, it constitutes the main prognostic factor in the majority of the cases. Because of its severe conditions and in some cases along with therapy, the gravity of the infection. However, it is not rare that an infection of an unexpected severity develops in a cancer patient whose tumor is well controlled. This means that the prognosis also depends on the nature of the added infection.

Some general factors have an unquestionable prognostic interest. Fever observed during irradiation of cancer of the uterus carries an unfavorable prognosis, even if its infectious origin is not proved (Van Herik, 1965). An important element is the age of the patient; an elderly patient tolerates less well than a younger one the additional burden of a severe infection. The type of infection may reflect a general impairment of the patient. In a series of hematologic malignancies reported by Aston *et al.* (1972), the mean survival of 7 months for all patients drops to one month for those presenting a herpes infection. The appearance of a banal herpes zoster in a Hodgkin's patient does not have a prognostic significance. On the contrary, a herpes virus complicated infection has a poor prognosis (Fig. 16). This fact is not due to a direct influence of infection on the patient's survival, but it means that infections are readily complicated in patients with advanced cancer, severe immune deficiency, and poor prognosis. For bacterial (Schimpff *et al.*, 1973) or parasitic (Walzer *et al.*, 1974) infections, the prognosis of the infection depends very often on the leukocytosis of the patient. The stage of the cancer also plays a role: If a complete remission has been obtained, the evolution is more favorable for bacterial (Atkinson *et al.*, 1974) or fungal (Bodey *et al.*, 1966) infections.

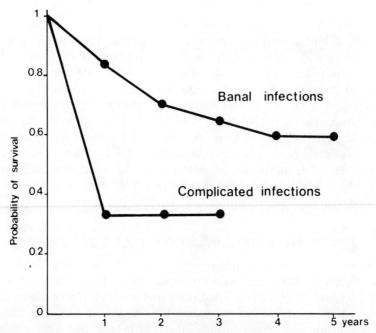

**Fig. 16.**  Actuarial survival of patients with hematologic neoplasm from the moment of herpes-virus skin infection, according to the type of infection (from Durand *et al.*, 1977).

Other factors depend directly on the type of infection, on the responsible microorganism and its sensitivity to treatment, and on the anatomo-clinical aspect of the infection. Thus, infections caused by Gram-negative bacteria, fungal infections, and pneumocystosis have, on the whole, a particular severity. The simultaneous association of several microorganisms aggravates the situation even more. A pneumocystosis, whose general prognosis is severe, may progress favorably while the patient dies of a supervening bacterial pneumonia (Rosen *et al.*, 1972). Even before anti-infectious treatment can be shown to be effective, an early diagnosis of the infection is essential in order to begin the most appropriate treatment. We have seen that the gravity of certain Gram-negative infections, capable of causing death in less than 48 hr, necessitates immediate antibiotic treatment, usually guided by the knowledge of the hospital microbial ecology (see Chapter 10). We have also seen that for the same microorganism, the infectious localization conditions the prognosis (see Chapter 5).

Finally, the well-known toxicity of anticancer chemotherapy should not overshadow the less frequent but sometimes severe toxicity of anti-infectious chemotherapy that may handicap the treatment of the infection or directly cause serious complications.

# Conclusion

The infectious problems that are actually confronted by doctors who treat cancer patients assume, as we have seen, a large importance which justifies the attention given to them and an indispensable collaboration between oncologists and infectious disease specialists. The necessary solutions needed to overcome present obstacles should, in the next few years, come from two directions: on the one hand the anti-infectious measures and on the other hand anticancer treatments.

Progress in the control of infectious agents is not a negligible approach. Some concern already exists about means which could be perfected: isolation of patients, (a subject of numerous and varied researches), is far from being completed and the increasing availability of efficacious leukocytes will also allow a better management of a deficiency which is often a turning point. Other treatments are only in the experimental stage or are only projects: manipulation of bacterial ecology in order to replace pathogenic flora with microorganisms less dangerous for the patient, use of new antibacterial agents or substances acting on the plasmids which are reponsible for resistance to antibiotics, and utilization of transfer factor.

However, these real difficulties often stress the insufficiency of anticancer treatments. Infections observed in cancer patients are regressing and will continue to do so in the measure where cancers can be more efficaciously treated, more often cured, for cancer cure definitively causes the disappearance of the majority of factors which favor infections. Infections would also regress if more efficacious treatments did not necessitate aplasia for the patient, i.e., if the difference between the efficacy and the toxicity (the therapeutic index) of the anticancer treatments increases.

Even before the application of treatment, an early diagnosis of a cancer can improve the situation. In fact, a tumor which is still limited and not very bulky is less likely to cause infection by local or general consequences which are still more minimal than for an advanced cancer. Moreover, the treatment of a small cancer is almost always simpler and more efficacious than that of a large tumor, which necessitates a more intensive and dangerous therapy for the patient.

161

In summary, infections actually reflect the insufficient oncological therapy. Their control depends on the quality of measures which contribute largely to the general results of the treatment. There is hope that a continuing decrease in their frequency will denote a sign of progress in the early detection of cancers, as well as in the comprehensive management of the disease and in a better control of its evolution.

# References

Abdallah, P. S., Mark, J. B. D., and Merigan, T. C. (1976): Diagnosis of cytomegalovirus pneumonia in compromised host. *Am J Med 61:326–332.*

Abell, C., and Holland, P. (1969): Acute toxoplasmosis complicating leukemia. Diagnosis by bone marrow aspiration. *Am J Dis Child 118:782–787.*

Ackerman, N. B., and Kronmueller, J. (1975): The importance of candida as an infectious agent. *Surg Gynecol Obstet 140:65–68.*

Adam, M., Morgan, O., Persaud, C., and Gibbs, W. (1973): Hyperinfection syndrome with Strongyloides stercoralis. *Br Med J 1:264–266.*

Adenis, L., Herpeau, J., Colpin, A., and Mouton, Y. (1975): Varicelle pulmonaire. *Nouv Presse Med 4:354.*

Adler, J. L., Burke, J. P., Martin, D. F., and Finland, M. (1971a): *Proteus* infections in a general hospital: I. Biochemical characteristics and antibiotics susceptibility of the organism. *Ann Intern Med 75:517–530.*

Adler, J. L., Burke, Martin, D. F., and Finland, M. (1971b): *Proteus* infections in a general hospital: II. Some clinical and epidemiological characteristics. *Ann Intern Med 75:531–536.*

Aisner, J., Schimpff, S. C., Bennett, J. E., Young, V. M., and Wiernik, P. H. (1976): Aspergillus infections in cancer patients. Association with fire-proofing materials in a new hospital. *J Am Med Assoc 235:411–412.*

Aisner, J., Schimpff, S. C., Sutherland, J. E., Young, V. M., and Wiernik, P. H. (1976): (1976): *Torulopsis glabrata* infections in patients with cancer. Increasing incidence and relationship to colonization. *Am J Med 61:23–28.*

Aisner, J., Sickles, E. A., Schimpff, S. C., Young, V. M., Greene, W.H., and Wiernik, P. H. (1974): *Torulopsis glabrata* pneumonitis in patients with cancer. Report of three cases. *J Am Med Assoc 230:584–585.*

Alavi, J. B., Root, R. K., Djerassi, I., Evans, A. E., Gluckman, S. J., MacGregor, R. R., Guerry, D., Schreiber, A. D., Shaw, J. M., Koch, P., and Cooper, R. A. (1977): A randomized clinical trial of granulocyte transfusions for infection in acute leukemia. *N Engl J Med 296:706–711.*

Alpern, R. J., and Dowell, V. R., Jr. (1969): *Clostridium septicum* infections and malignancy. *J Am Med Assoc 209:385–388.*

Amblard, P., Schaerer, R., Sotto, J. J., Martel, J., Bensa, J. C., and Fillon, J. P. (1973): Les manifestations cutanées de la maladie de Hodgkin. A propos de l'étude systématique de 94 sujets porteurs de cette affection. *Sem Hop Paris 49:3073–3078.*

Ambrus, J. L., Ambrus, C. M., Mink, I. B., and Pickren, J. W. (1975): Causes of death in cancer patients. *J Med Soc NY 6:61–64.*

Amiel, J. L., Sekiguchi, M., Daguet, G., Garattini, S., and Palma, V. (1967): Etude de l'effet immunodépresseur des composés chimiques utilisés en chimiothérapie anticancéreuse. *Eur J Cancer 3:47–65.*

163

Andersen, B., Korner, B., and Ostergaard, A. H. (1972): Topical ampicillin against wound infection after colorectal surgery. *Ann Surg 176:129–132.*

Anderson, T., Schein, P. S., Jencks, J. A., and Binder, R. A. (1974): The nitroblue tetrazolium (NBT) dye test in determining fever source in lymphoma. *Cancer 34:705–710.*

Anner, R. M., Nydegger, U., Lambert, P. H., and Miescher, P. A. (1975): Intérêt et limites du test au nitrobleu de tétrazolium dans divers états fébriles. *Sem Hop Paris 51:1701–1705.*

Armengaud, M., Auvergnat, J. C., Guiraud, R., Le Net, R., and Simon, J. (1976): Intérêt des polynucléaires marqués dans le dépistage précoce d'une suppuration. *Med Mal Infect 6:201–206.*

Armstrong, D. (1973): Infectious complications in cancer patients treated with chemical immunosuppressive agents. *Transplant Proc 5:1245–1248.*

Armstrong, D. (1976): Interstitial pneumonia in the immunosuppressed patient. *Transplant Proc 8:657–661.*

Arnaud, J. P., Prat, J. J., Griscelli, C., Gentilini, M., and Nezelof, C. (1976): Le diagnostic de la pneumonie à Pneumocystis carinii par l'immunofluorescence indirecte. Technique, intérèt et limites do le méthode. *Nouv Presse Med 5:2607–2610.*

Aronson, M. D., Phillips, C. F., Gump, D. W., Albertini, R. J., and Phillips, C. A. (1976): Vidarabine therapy for severe virus infections. *J Am Med Assoc 235:1339–1342.*

Asada, T. (1974): Treatment of human cancer with mumps virus. *Cancer 34:1907–1928.*

Aston, D. L., Cohen, A., and Spindler, M. A. (1972): Herpes virus homini infection in patients with myeloproliferative and lymphoproliferative disorders. *Br Med J 4:462–465.*

Athanassiades, S., Deligeorge, H., Kalachanis, N., and Paraskevas, G. (1973): Pathologic changes in the gastroduodenal mucosa after intra-arterial infusion of 5-fluorouracil. *Am J Surg 126:319–321.*

Atkinson, K., Kay, H. E., and McElwain, T. J. (1974): Fever in the neutropenic patient. *Br Med J 3:160–161.*

Atkinson, K., Kay, H. E., and McElwain, T. J. (1974): Septicaemia in the neutropenic patients. *Br Med J 3:244–247.*

Aubertin, E., and Aubertin, J. (1963): Fièvre au long cours, manifestations d'un processus malin latent. *Gaz Hop Paris 135, 751–763.*

Aubertin, J., Legendre, P., Merlet, M., Issanchou, A. M., Lacut, J. Y., and Leng, B. 1977): Le risque infectieux au cours des aplasies médullaires. *Bordeaux Med 10:255–263.*

Aubertin, J., and Leng, B. (1973): Les candidoses. *Encycl Med Chir 8125 A10.*

Aubertin, J., Leng, B., Lacut, J. Y., and Buy, E. (1974): Les fièvres prolongées. Etude critique de 400 observations. *Bordeaux Med 7:1291–1308.*

Aubertin, J., Leng, B., Lacut, J. Y., Le Gall, F., and Boget, J. C. (1972): Les infections acquises à cytomégalovirus. Etude critique. *Bordeaux Med 5:2727–2741.*

Audran, R. (1970): Notions actuelles concernant de complément. *Rev Eur Et Clin Biol 15:610–637.*

Aungst, C. W., Sokal, J. E., and Jager, B. V. (1975): Complication of BCG vaccinations in neoplastic disease. *Ann Intern Med 82:666–669.*

Baehner, R. L., Neiburger, R. G., Johnson, D. E., and Murrmann, S. M. (1973): Transient bactericidal defect of peripheral blood lymphocytes from children with acute leukemia receiving craniospinal irradiation. *N Engl J Med 289:1209–1213.*

Barlotta, F. M., Ochoa, M., Jr., Neu, H. C., and Ultmann, J. E. (1969): Toxoplasmosis, lymphoma or both. *Ann Intern Med 70:517–528.*

Barnes, E. W., Farmer, A., Penhale, W. J., Irvine, W. J., Roscoe, P., and Horne, N. W. (1975): Phytohemagglutinin-induced lymphocyte transformation in newly presenting patients with primary carcinoma of the lung. *Cancer 36:187–193.*

Barnett, R. N., Hull, J. G., Vortel, V., and Schwarz, J. (1969): Pneumocystis carinii in lymph nodes and spleen. *Arch Pathol 88:175–180.*

Bartrum, R. J., Watnick, M., and Herman, P. G. (1973): Roentgenographic finding in pulmonary mucormycosis. *Am J Roentgenol Radium Ther Nucl Med 117:810–815.*

Bastin, R., and Frottier, J. (1969): Une difficulté de tous les jours en pathologie infectieuse, l'interprétation des résultats de séro-diagnostic. *Rev Med Paris 10:1207–1215.*

Bastin, R., Pechere, J. C., Frottier, J., Calamy, G., and Vilde, J. L. (1971): Résultats thérapeutiques des associations d'antibiotiques bactéricides dans les infections septicémiques. *Pathol Biol 19:585–591.*

Beaugrand, M., Renoux, M., Molas, G., Altman, J. J., and Bernades, P. (1976): Colite aigué à cytomégalovirus chez des sujets immunodeprimes. Presentation de deux cas. *Arch Fr Mal App Dig 65:189–196.*

Beauvais, B., Garin, J. F., Larivière, M., and Languillat, G. (1976): Toxoplasmose et leucémie myéloïde chronique. *Nouv Rev Fr Hematol 16:169–184.*

Bennett, J. E. (1974): Chemotherapy of systemic mycoses. *N Engl J. Med 290:30–32 and 320–323.*

Ben-Shoshan, M., Gius, J. A., and Smith, I. M. (1971): Exploratory laparotomy for fever of unknown origin. *Surg Gynecol Obstet 132:994–996.*

Bentegeat, J., Boisseau, M., Chauvergne, J., Hoerni, B., De Joigny, C., Le Treut, A., Mandoul, R., Simon, G., Verdaguer, S., and Mesnier, F. (1969): Toxoplasmose et lymphoréticulopathies malignes. *Bordeaux Med 2:1169–1179.*

Berenyi, M. R., Straus, B., and Avila, L. (1975): T rosettes in alcoholic cirrhosis of the liver. *J Am Med Assoc 232:44–46.*

Bernadou, A., Nutini, M. T., Blanc, C. M., Smadja, R., and Bousser, J. (1971): L'immunité cellulaire dans la leucémie lymphoïde chronique (Etude de 61 cas). *Nouv Rev Fr Hematol 11:470–475.*

Bernard, J. (1967): Leucopénies et leucocytoses modérées. *Actual Hematol 1:3–13.*

Bernard, J., Boiron, M., Levy, J. P., Ripault, J., and Desmonts, G. (1962). Toxoplasmose généralisée associèe à une leucémie aiguë. *Nouv Rev Fr Hematol 2:910–914.*

Berry, D. H., Pullen, J., George, S., Vietti, T. J., Sullivan, M. P., and Fernbach, D. (1975): Comparison of prednisolone, vincristine, methotrexate and 6-mercaptopurine vs. vincristine and prednisone induction therapy in childhood acute leukemia. *Cancer 36:98–102.*

Berthelot, P., Sicot, C., Benhamou, J. P., and Fauvert, R. (1965): Les hépatites médicamenteuses. II. Etude analytique des médicaments responsables. *Rev Fr Et Clin Biol 10:140–179.*

Bientz, M., and Rochemaure, J. (1973): Les pneumopathies à pneumocystis carinii de l'adulte. *Poumon coeur 19:5–12.*

Bindschadler, D. D., and Bennett, J. E. (1968): Serology of human cryptococcosis. *Ann Intern Med 69:45–52.*

Bjorgen, J. E., and Gold, L. H. A. (1977): Computed tomographic appearance of methotrexate-induced necrotizing leukoencephalopathy. *Radiology 122:377–378.*

Bjorn-Hansen, R., and Hagen, S. (1970): Abdominal lymphography: A study with special reference to the individual variations in dosage of contrast medium. *Am J Roentgenol Radium Ther Nucl Med 110:846–852*.

Block, J. B., Haynes, H. A., Thomson, W. L., and Neiman, P. E. (1969): Delayed hypersensitivity in chronic lymphocytic leukemia. *J Natl Cancer Inst 42:973–980*.

Bloomfield, C. D., and Kennedy, B. J. (1974): Cephalothin, carbenicillin and gentamicin combination therapy for febrile patients with acute non-lymphocytic leukemia. *Cancer 34:431–437*.

Bloomfield, N., Gordon, M. S., and Elmendorf, D. F., Jr. (1963): Detection of Cryptococcus neoformans antigen in body fluids by latex particle agglutination. *Proc Soc Exp Biol Med 114:64–67*.

Bodel, P. (1974): Tumors and fever. *Ann NY Acad Sci 230:6–13*.

Bodel, P., and Atkins, E. (1967): Release of endogenous pyrogen by human monocytes. *N Engl J Med 276:1002–1008*.

Bodey, G., McKelvey, F., and Karon, M. (1964): Chicken pox in leukemic patients. Factors in prognosis. *Pediatrics 34:562–567*.

Bodey, G. P. (1966): Fungal infections complicating acute leukemia. *J Chron Dis 19:667–687*.

Bodey, G. P. (1973): Patient isolation units for cancer patients treated with chemical immunosuppressive agents. *Transplant Proc 5:1279–1284*.

Bodey, G. P., Buckley, M., Sathe, Y. S., and Freireich, E. I. (1966): Quantitative relationships between circulating leucocytes and infection in patients with acute leukemia. *Ann Intern Med 64:328–340*.

Bodey, G. P., DeJongh, D., Isassi, A., and Freireich, E. J. (1969): Hypersplenism due to disseminated candidiasis in a patient with acute leukemia. *Cancer 24:417–420*.

Bodey, G. P., Middleman, E., Umsawadi, T., and Rodriguez, V. (1972): Infections in cancer patients. Results with gentamicin sulfate therapy. *Cancer 29:1697–1701*.

Bodey, G. P., and Rodriguez, V. (1973): Advances in the management of *Pseudomonas aeruginosa* infections in cancer patients. *Eur J. Cancer 9:435–441*.

Bodey, G. P., and Rodriguez, V. (1975): Infections in cancer patients in a protected environment. Prophylactic antibiotic program. *Am J Med 59:497–504*.

Bodey, G. P., Rodriguez, V., and Luce, J. K. (1969): Carbenicillin therapy of gram negative bacilli infections. *Am J Med Sci 257:408–414*.

Bodey, G. P., Rodriguez, V., and Smith, J. P. (1970): Serratia sp. infections in cancer patients. *Cancer 25:199–205*.

Bodey,, G. P., Watson, P., Cooper, C., and Freireich, E. J. (1971): Protected environments: Units for the cancer patients. *Cancer 21:215–219*.

Bodey, G. P., Whitecar, J. P., Middleman, E., and Rodriguez, V. (1971): Carbenicillin therapy of Pseudomonas infections. *J Am Med Assoc 218:62–66*.

Boetcher, D. A., and Leonard, E. J. (1974): Abnormal monocyte chemotatic response in cancer patients. *J Natl Cancer Inst 52:1091–1099*.

Boggs, D. R. (1974): Transfusion of neutrophils as prevention or treatment of infections in patients with neutropenia. *N Engl J Med 290:1055–1062*.

Boggs, D. R. (1977): Neutrophil in the blood bank. *N Engl J Med 296:748–750*.

Boggs, D. R., and Frei, E., III. (1960): Clinical studies of fever and infection in cancer. *Cancer 13:1240–1253*.

Boggs, D. R., Williams, A. F., and Howell, A., Jr. (1961): Thrush in malignant neoplastic disease. *Arch Intern Med 107:354–360*.

Bolton, P. M., Mander, A. M., Davidson, J. M., James, S. L., Newcombe, R. G., and

Hughes, L. E. (1975): Cellular immunity in cancer: comparison of delayed hypersensitivity skin tests in three common cancers. *Br Med J 3:18–20.*

Bordos D. C., Baker, R. R., and Cameron, J. L. (1974): An evaluation of palliative abdominoperineal resection for carcinoma of the rectum. *Surg Gynecol Obstet 139:731–733.*

Bourgeaux, C., Trepo, C., Bordes, M., Sizaret, P., Martin, F., Sananes, R., Sepetjian, M., and Klepping, C. (1975): Etude de l'antigène Australia dans les cancers primitifs du foie. Ses rapports avec l'alpha-foetoprotein. *Biol gastroenterol 6:133–137.*

Brazinsky, J. H., and Phillips, J. E. (1969): Pneumocystis pneumonia transmission between patients with lymphoma. *J Am Med Assoc 209:1527.*

Breitfeld, V., Yashida, Y., Sherman, F. E., Odagiri, K., and Yunis, E. J. (1973): Fatal measles infection in children with leukemia. *Lab Invest 28:279–291.*

Brisou, B., Hauteville, D., De Saint-Julien, J., Pholoppe, P. E., and Chamfeuil, R. (1975): Les septicémies humaines à Aeromonas hydrophila. Etude clinique et bactériologique d'un cas. *Med Mal Infect 5:248–253.*

Brooks, W. H., Netsky, M. G., Normansell, D. E., and Horwitz, D. A. (1972): Depressed cell-mediated immunity in patients with primary intracranial tumors. *J Exp Med 136:1631–1647.*

Brun, F. E. (1971): Die kutan-allergische Spätreaktion auf 2,4-Dinitrochlorbenzol bei Krebspatienten unter zytostatischer Chemotherapie. *Schweiz Med Wschr 101:1235–1243.*

Buckman, R., and Wiltshaw, E. (1976): Progressive multifocal leucoencephalopathy successfully treated with cytosine arabinoside. *Brit J Haemat 34:153–155.*

Burdick, J. F., Wells, S. A., Jr., and Herberman, R. B. (1975): Immunologic evaluation of patients with cancer by delayed hypersensitivity reactions. *Surg Gynecol Obstet 141:779–794.*

Burke, P. S., and Coltman, C. A., Jr. (1971): Multiple pulmonary aspergillomas in acute leukemias. *Cancer 28:1289–1292.*

Burkitt, D. P., and Wright, D. H. (1970): *Burkitt's Lymphoma.* Livingstone, London, vol. 1.

Bussel, A., Benbunan, M., Tanzer, J., and Boiron, M. (1971): Transfusions de leucocytes au cours des aplasies après chimiothérapie antileucémique. *Actual Hematol 5:169–180.*

Bussel, A., Montant, G., Danon, F., and Perol, Y. (1975): Septicémies à cytomégalovirus et hémopathies malignes. A propos de 33 observations. *Actual Hematol 9:134–149.*

Cady, B., and Clifton, E. E. (1967): Empyema and survival following surgery for bronchogenic carcinoma. *J Thorac Cardiovasc Surg 53:102–108.*

Cale, D. C., Reynolds, H. Y., Pennington, J. E., Elin, R. J., and Herzig, P. P. (1976): Experimental Pseudomonas pneumonia in leukopenic dogs: comparison of therapy with antibiotics and granulocyte transfusions. *Blood 47:869–876.*

Callerame, M. L., and Nadel, M. (1966): Pneumocystis carinii pneumonia in two adults with multiple myeloma. *Am J Clin Pathol 45:258–263.*

Camilleri, J. P., and Diebold, J. (1972): Complications pulmonaires terminales des leucoses aiguës. *Pathol Eur 7:83–93.*

Campbell, G. D. (1966): Primary pulmonary cryptococcosis. *Am Rev Resp Dis 94:236–243.*

Campbell, P. C. (1965): Large doses of penicillin in the prevention of surgical wound infection. *Lancet 2:805–810.*

Cangir, A., Sullivan, M. P., Sutow, W. W., and Taylor, G. (1967): Cytomegalo-virus syndrome in children with acute leukemia. Treatment with floxurudine. *J Am Med Assoc 201:612–615.*

Cappel, R., Salhadin, A., and Klastersky, J. (1973): Apport de la ponction trans-trachéale dans le diagnostic des infections et des néoplasies pulmonaires. Aspects bactériologiques, virologiques et cytologiques sur un relevé de 124 patients. *Nouv Presse Med 2:787–790.*

Carey, R. M., Kimball, A. C., Armstrong, D. A., and Lieberman, P. H. (1973): Toxoplasmosis. Clinical experience in a cancer hospital. *Am J Med 54:30–38.*

Carl, W., Schaaf, N. G., and Chen, T. Y. (1972): Oral care of patients irradiated for cancer of the head and neck. *Cancer 30:448–453.*

Carnovale, R., Zornoza, J., Goldman, A. M., and Luna, M. (1977): Pulmonary alveolar proteinosis: Its association with hematologic malignancy and lymphoma. *Radiology 122:303–306.*

Carroll, B. A., Lane, B., Norman, D., and Enzmann, D. (1977): Diagnosis of progressive multifocal leukoencephalopathy by computed tomography. *Radiology 122:137–141.*

Casazza, A. R., Duvall, C. P., and Carbone, P. P. (1966): Summary of infectious complications occurring in patients with Hodgkin's disease. *Cancer Res 26:1290–1296.*

Cassi, E., and Visca, U. (1966): Toxoplasmosi linfoghiandolare e linforgranuloma di Hodgkin. *Policlinico 73:1225–1234.*

Catalano, L. W., Jr., and Goldman, J. M. (1972): Antibody to herpes virus hominis types 1 and 2 in patients with Hodgkin's disease and carcinoma of the nasopharynx. *Cancer 29:597–602.*

Catalona, W. J., and Chretien, P. B. (1973): Abnormalities in quantitative dinitro-chlorobenzene sensitization in cancer patients: Correlation with tumor stage and histology. *Cancer 31:353–356.*

Catalona, W. J., Sample, W. F., and Chretien, P. B.(1973): Lymphocyte reactivity in cancer patients: Correlation with tumor histology and clinical stage. *Cancer 31:65–71.*

Caul, E. O., Dickinson, V. A., Roome, A. P., Mott, M. G., and Stevenson, P. A. (1972): Cytomegalovirus infections in leukaemic children. *Int J Cancer 10:213–220.*

Chang, W. W. L., and Buerger, L. (1964): Disseminated geotrichosis. Case report. *Arch Intern Med 113:356–360.*

Chauvergne, J., Hoerni, B., Hoerni-Simon, G., Durand, M., and Lagarde, C. (1973): Chimiothérapie de la maladie de Hodgkin associant procarbazine, vinblastine, cyclophosphamide et méthyl-prednisolone. Analyse d'une série de 124 cures. *Z Krebsforsch 80:179–188.*

Chauvergne, J., Meugé, C., Boisseau, M., and Hoerni, B. (1969): Lymphoréti-culopathie maligne et toxoplasmose. *Sem Hop Paris 45:2816–2821.*

Check, J. H., Damsker, J. I., Brady, L. W., and O'Neill, E. A. (1973): Effect of radiation therapy on mumps-delayed type hypersensitivity reaction in lymphoma and carcinoma patients. *Cancer 32:580–584.*

Chen, T. Y., and Webster, J. H. (1974): Oral monilia study on patients with head and neck cancer during radiotherapy. *Cancer 34:246–249.*

Ch'ien, L. T., Whitley, R. J., Alford, C. A., Galasso, G. J., and the Collaborative Study Group (1976): Adenosine arabinoside for therapy of herpes-zoster in immunosuppressed patients: Preliminary results of a collaborative study. *J. Infect Dis 133:A184–A191.*

Chilcote, R. R., Baehner, R. L., Hammond, D., and the Investigators and Special Studies Committee of the Children's Cancer Study Group (1976): Septicemia and meningitis in children splenectomized for Hodgkin's disease. *N Engl J Med* 295:798–800.

Clement, J. A., and Kramer, S. (1974): Immunocompetence in patients with solid tumors undergoing cobalt 60 irradiation. *Cancer* 34:193–196.

Cochran, A. J., Spilg, W. G. S., Mackie, R. M., and Thomas, C. E. (1972): Post operative depression of tumour-directed cell-mediated immunity in patients with malignant disease. *Br Med J* 4:67–70.

Cohen, M. H., Creaven, P. J., Fossieck, B. E., Johnston, A. V., and Williams, C. L. (1976): Effect of oral prophylactic broad spectrum non absorbable antibiotics on the gastrointestinal absorption of nutrients and methotrexate in small cell bronchogenic carcinoma patients. *Cancer* 38:1556–1559.

Cohen, M. L., Weiss, E. B., and Monaco, A. P. (1971): Successful treatment of Pneumocystis carinii and Nocardia asteroides in a renal transplant patient. *Am J Med* 50:269–276.

Conomy, J. P., Beard, S., Matsumoto, H., and Roessmann, V. (1974): Cytarabine treatment of progressive multifocal leukoencephalopathy. Clinical course and detection of virus like particles after antiviral chemotherapy. *J Am Med Assoc* 229:1313–1316.

Constantopoulos, A., Likhite, V., Crosby, W. H., and Najjar, V. A. (1973): Phagocytic activity of the leukemic cell and its response to the phagocystosis stimulating tetrapeptide, tuftsin. *Cancer Res* 33:1230–1234.

Coonrod, J. D., and Rytel, M. W. (1972): Determination of etiology of bacterial meningitis by counterimmunoelectrophoresis. *Lancet* 1:1154–1157.

Copeland, E. M., III, MacFadyen, B. V., Jr., McGown, C., and Dudrick, S.J. (1974): The use of hyperalimentation in patients with potential sepsis. *Surg Gynecol Obstet* 138:377–380.

Cox, F., and Hughes, W. T. (1974): Disseminated histoplasmosis and childhood leukemia. *Cancer* 33:1127–1133.

Cox, F., and Hughes, W. T. (1975): The value of isolation procedures for cytomegalovirus infections in children with leukemia. *Cancer* 36:1158–1161.

Craddock, P. R., Yawata, Y., Vansanten, L., Gilberstadt, S., Silvis, S., and Jacob, H. S. (1974): Acquired phagocyte dysfunction. A complication of the hypophosphatemia of parenteral hyperalimentation. *N Engl J Med* 290:1403–1407.

Crout, J. E., Hepburn, B., and Ritts, R. E., Jr. (1975): Suppression of lymphocyte transformation after aspirin ingestion. *N Engl J Med* 292:221–223.

Crowther, D. (1973): Immunological aspects, in *Hodgkin's Disease,* D. Smithers (Ed.), Livingstone, London, vol. 1, pp. 86–103.

Dale, D. C., Reynolds, H. Y., Pennington, J. E., Elin, R. J., and Herzig, G. P. (1976): Experimental Pseudomonas pneumonia in leukopenic dogs: Comparison of therapy with antibiotics and granulocyte transfusions. *Blood* 47:869–876.

Dao, C. (1971): Les complications infectieuses des leucémies aiguës: prévention par une antibiothérapie générale; résultats d'une étude prospective portant sur 75 dossiers. Détermination de l'origine exogène ou endogène des germes de surinfection. Thèse, Paris.

Dao, C. (1973): Aspects cliniques, hématologiques, virologiques des affections à cytomégalovirus. *Sem Hop Paris* 49:273–278.

Dao, C. (1975): Infections des agranulocytoses et leur traitement. *Sem Hosp Paris* 51:677–684.

Dao, C., Gerbal, R., Bernadou, A., Zittoun, R., Bilksi-Pasquier, G., and Bousser, J. (1973): Prévention des complications infectieuses des leucémies aiguës: place de l'antibiothérapie générale et intestinale. *Sem Hop Paris 49:1067–1076.*

Davis C. M., Vandersarl, J. V., Coltman, C. A. (1973): Failure of cytarabine in varicella-zoster infections. *J Am Med Assoc 224:122–123.*

Dayan, A. D., Bhatti, I., and Gostling, J. V. T. (1967): Encephalitis due to herpes simplex in a patient with treated carcinoma of the uterus. *Neurology (Minneap) 17:609–613.*

Dean, M. M., and Post, R. M. (1967): Fatal infection with Aeromonas hydrophila in a patient with acute myelogenous leukemia. *Ann Intern Med 66:1177–1179.*

Debusscher, L., Thiry, L., and Klastersky, J. (1972): Bacterial colonization of the respiratory tract in hospitalized patients with malignant diseases. *Rev Eur Et Clin Biol 17:179–184.*

Deconti, R. C., Kaplan, S. R., Papac, R. J., and Calabresi, P. (1973): Continuous intravenous infusions of 5-fluoro-2'-deoxyuridine in the treatment of solid tumors. *Cancer 31:894–898.*

Deinard A. S., Fortuny, I. E., Theologides, A., Anderson, G. L., Boen, J., and Kennedy, B. J. (1974): Studies on the neutropenia of cancer chemotherapy. *Cancer 33:1210–1218.*

Delarue, J., Diebold, J., Camilleri, J. P., Reynes, M., and Bousser, M. G. (1969): Les hémopathies avec protéinose alvéolaire pulmonaire. Revue des cas publiés à propos d'une nouvelle observation. *Arch Anat Pathol 17:71–78.*

Deresinski, S. C., and Stevens, D. A. (1974): Conidiomycosis in compromised hosts. *Medicine 54:377–395.*

Desser, R. K., and Ultmann, J. E. (1972): Risk of severe infection in patients with Hodgkin's disease or lymphoma after diagnostic laparotomy and splenectomy. *Ann Intern Med 77:143–146.*

De-Thé, G., Epstein, M. A., and Hausen, H. (1975): *Oncogenesis and Herpesviruses.* IARC, Lyon.

DeVita, V. T., Jr., Emmer, M., Levine, A., Jacobs, B., and Berard, C. (1969): *Pneumoycystis carinii* pneumonia: successful diagnosis and treatment of two patients with associated malignant processes. *N Engl J Med 280:287–291.*

DeVita, V. T., Jr., and Young, R. C. (1973): Infection and cancer: Old friends. *Ann Intern Med 79:577–579.*

Diamond, R. D., and Bennett, J. E. (1974): Prognostic factors in cryptococcal meningitis. A study in 111 cases. *Ann Intern Med 80:176–181.*

Diaz-Jouanen, E., Strickland, R. G., and Williams, R. C., Jr. (1975): Studies of human lymphocytes in the newborn and the aged. *Am J Med 58:620–628.*

Dietrich, M., Rasche, H., Rommel, K., and Hochappel, G. (1973): Antimicrobial therapy as a part of the decontamination procedures for patients with acute leukemia. *Eur J Cancer 9:443–447.*

Diggs, C. M., Eskenasy, G. M., Sutherland, J. C., and Wiernik, P. H. (1976): Fungal infections of muscle in acute leukemia. *Cancer 38:1771–1772.*

Dmochowski, L. (1960): Viruses and tumors in the light of electron microscope studies. A review. *Cancer Res 20:977–1015.*

Dmochowski, L., Yumoto, T., Grey, C. E., Hales, R. L., Langford, P. L., Taylor, H. G., Freireich, E. J., Shullenberger, C. C., Shively, J. A., and Howe, C. D. (1967): Electron microscopic studies of human leukemia and lymphoma. *Cancer 20:760–777.*

Domart, A., Hazard, J., Labram, C., Husson, R., and Portos, J. L. (1964): Varicelle hémorragique avec pneumopathie chez un adulte traité par la delta-cortisone pour leucose aiguë. *Presse Med 72:235–238.*

Donaldson, S. S., Moore, M. R., Rosenberg, S. A., and Vasti, K. L. (1972): Occurrence of post splenectomy bacteriemia among patients with and without lymphoma. *N Engl J Med 287:69–71.*

Doppman, J. L., Geelhoed, G. W., and DeVita, V. T. (1975). Atypical radiographic features in *Pneumocystis carinii* pneumonia. *Radiology 114:39–44.*

Dorff, G. J., Coonrod, J. D., and Rytel, M. W. (1971): Detection by immunoelectrophoresis of antigen in sera of patients with pneumococcal bacteraemia. *Lancet 1:578–579.*

Dorfman, R. F., and Remington, J. S. (1973): Value of lymph-node biopsy in the diagnosis of acute acquired toxoplasmosis. *N Engl J Med 289:878–881.*

Drew, W. L., Finley, T. N., Mintz, L., and Klein, H. Z. (1974): Diagnosis of *Pneumocystis carinii* pneumonia by bronchopulmonary lavage. *J Am Med Assoc 230:713–715.*

Dreyfus, B. (1966): Confrontations thérapeutiques. I. Zona tenace et leucémie lymphoïde avec hypogammaglobulinémie. *Nouv Rev Fr Hematol 6:505–507.*

Dubin, I. N. (1947): The poverty of the immunological mechanism in patients with Hodgkin's disease. *Ann Intern Med 27:898–913.*

Dupuy J. M., Kourilsky, F. M., Fradelizzi, D., Feingold, N., Jacquillat, C., Bernard, J., and Dausset J. (1971): Depression of immunologic reactivity of patients with acute leukemia. *Cancer 27:323–331.*

Durand, M., Chauvergne, J., and Hoerni, B. (1972): Aspects immunologiques des complications infectieuses de la maladie de Hodgkin. *Bordeaux Med 5:1295–1298.*

Durand, M., Hoerni, B., Lacut, P. Y., and Chauvergne, J. (1974): Infection et fièvre en cancérologie médicale. Enquête épidémiologique portant sur 1162 malades. *Bordeaux Med 7:1309–1318.*

Durand, M., Hoerni, B., Lacut, J. Y., Hoerni-Simon, G., and Chauvergne, J. (1975): Complications infectieuses des lymphomes malins. Bilan de 411 observations observées chez 629 malades. *Ann Med Interne 126:251–256.*

Durand, M., Hoerni-Simon, G., Chauvergue, J., and Hoerni, B. (1974): Antibiothérapie préventive systématique chez les cancéreux leucopéniques. Résultats d'une étude contrôlée portant sur 50 malades. *Bordeaux Med 7:1405–1408.*

Durand, M., Jaubert, D., Lacut, J. Y., and Hoerni-Simon, G. (1976): La listériose neuroméningée au cours des hémopathies malignes. A propos d'une observation. Revue de la littérature. *Bordeaux Med 9:1209–1218.*

Durand, M., Reiffers, J., Hoerni-Simon, G., Chauvergne, J., and Hoerni, B. (1976): Infections cutanées à herpesvirus et hémopathies malignes. Epidémiologie. *Bull Cancer 6:433–440.*

Durand, M., Reiffers, J., Hoerni-Simon, G., Lacut, J. Y., and Hoerni, B. (1977). Infections cutanées à herpesvirus et hémopathies malignes. Clinique et évolution. *Bordeaux Med 10:565–569.*

Edwards, L. D., and Digioia, R. (1976): Infections in splenectomized patients. A study of 131 patients. *Scand J Infect Dis 8:255–261.*

Eickhoff, T. C. (1973): Infectious complications in renal transplant recipients. *Transplant Proc 5:1233–1238.*

Einzig, S., Hong, R., and Sharp, A. L. (1969): Successful treatment of pneumocystis carinii in an immunologically deficient acute lymphatic leukemia patient. *Cancer 23:658–662.*

Enck, R. E., and Bennett, J. M. (1976): Isolation of Haemophilus aphrophilus from an adult with acute leukemia. *J Clin Microbiol 4:194–195.*

E.O.R.T.C. (Cooperative group for Leukaemia and Reticulocytoses) (1972): Bleomycin in the reticuloses. *Br Med J 1:285–286.*

Epstein, E. H., Levin, D. L., Croft, J. D., and Lutzner, M. A. (1972): Mycosis fungoides .Survival, prognostis features, response to therapy and autopsy findings. *Medicine Balt 15:61–72.*

Epstein, L. B., and Salmon, S. E. (1974): The production of interferon by malignant plasmacells from patients with multiple myeloma. *J Immunol 112:1131–1138.*

Epstein, R. B., Clift, R. A., and Thomas, E. D. (1969): The effect of leukocyte transfusions on experimental bacteremia in the dog. *Blood 34:782–790.*

Eras, P., Goldstein, M. J., and Sherlock, P. (1972): Candida infection of the gastrointestinal tract. *Medicine 51:367–379.*

Ervin, F. R., and Bullock, W. E. (1976): Clinical and pharmacological studies of ticarcillin in Gram negative infections. *Antimicrob Agents Chemother 9:94–101.*

Escourolle, R., Hauw, J. J., Signoret, J. L., and Lhermitte, F. (1973): Leucoencéphalopathie multifocale progressive au cours d'une tuberculose ganglionnaire. *Nouv Presse Med 2:1277–1281.*

Esterly, J. (1968): *Pneumocystis carinii* in lung of adults at autopsy. *Am Rev Resp Dis 97:935–937.*

Esterly, J. A., and Warner, N. E. (1965): Pneumocystis carinii pneumonia. 12 cases in patients with neoplastic lymphoreticular disease. *Arch Pathol Chicago 80:433–441.*

Everson, T. C., and Cole, W. H. (1966): *Spontaneous Regression of Cancer.* Saunders, Philadelphia.

Fass, R. J., and Perkins, R. L. (1971): 5-Fluorocytosine in the treatment of cryptococcal and candida mycoses. *Ann Intern Med 74:535–539.*

Fauconnier, B. (1972): Moyens de défense de l'organisme contre les infections à virus. *Nouv Presse Med 1:13–118.*

Feld, R., Bodey, G. P., and Gröschel, D. (1976): Mycobacteriosis in patients with malignant disease. *Arch Intern Med 136:67–70.*

Feldman, S., and Cox, F. (1976): Viral infections and haematological malignancies. *Clin Haematol 5:311–328.*

Feldman, S., Webster, R. G., and Sugg, M. (1977): Influenza in children and young adults with cancer. *Cancer 39:350–353.*

Fischer, R., Becker, H. R., Joist, J. H., and Tismer, R. (1969): Pneumocystis-carinii—Pneumonie beim Erwachsenen. *Dtsch Med Wschr 94:2135–2140.*

Fishman, L. S., and Armstrong, D. (1972): Pseudomonas aeruginosa bacteremia in patients with neoplastic diseases. *Cancer 30:764–773.*

Flandring, G., Daniel, M. T., Fourcade, M., and Chelloul, N. (1973): Leucémie à "tricholeucocyte" (hairy cell leukemia), étude clinique et cytologique de 55 observations. *Nouv Rev Fr Hematol 13:609–640.*

Folland, D., Armstrong, D., Seides, S., and Blevins, A. (1974): Pneumococcal bacteremia in patients with neoplastic disease. *Cancer 33:845–849.*

Forkner, C. C., Jr., Frei, E., III, Edgcomb, J. H., and Utz, J. P. (1958): Pseudomonas septicemia. Observations of twenty-three cases. *Am J Med 24:877–888.*

Forrest, J. V. (1972): Radiographic findings in Pneumocystis carinii pneumonia. *Radiology 103:539–544.*

Fortuny, I. E., Tempero, K. F., and Amsden, T. W. (1970): Pneumocystis carinii pneumonia diagnosed from sputum and successfully treated with pentamidine isethionate. *Cancer 26:911–913.*

Foy, H. M., Ochs, H., Davis, S. D., Kenny, G. E., and Luce, R. R. (1973): Mycoplasma pneumoniae infections in patients with immunodeficiency syndromes: Report of four cases. *J Infect Dis 127:388–393.*

Freckman, H. R. (1971): Chemotherapy for metastatic colorectal liver carcinoma by intra-aortic infusion. *Cancer 28:1152–1160.*

Frei, E., III, Levin, R. H., Bodey, G. P., Morse, E. E., and Freireich, E. J. (1965): The nature and control of infections in patients with acute leukemia. *Cancer Res 25:1511–1515.*

Gaiffe, M., Herzog, F., and Schweisguth, O. (1976): Efficacité préventive et curative du sérum de convalescent de zona et de varicelle chez les enfants à haut risque. *Nouv Presse Med 5:1285–1288.*

Galbraith, R. M., Eddleston, A. L. W. F., Williams, R., Zuckerman, A. J., and Bagshawe, K. D. (1975): Fulminant hepatic failure in leukaemia and choriocarcinoma related to withdrawal of cytotoxic drug therapy. *Lancet 2:528–530.*

Gaya, H., Tattersall, M. H. N., Hutchinson, R. M., and Spiers, A. S. D. (1973): Changing patterns of infection in cancer patients. *Eur J Cancer 9:401–406.*

Geelhoed, G. W., and Ketcham, A. S. (1973): *Pseudomonas* meningitis complicating radical resection for radiorecurrent cancer of paranasal sinuses: Report of two patients successfully treated with intrathecal polymyxin. *J Surg Oncol 5:365–374.*

Geiser, C. F., Bishop, Y., Myers, M. Jaffe, N., and Yankee, R. (1975): Prophylaxis of varicella in children with neoplastic disease: Comparative results with zoster immune plasma and gamma globulin. *Cancer Phila. 35:1027–1030.*

Gergovich, F. G., Richman, S. P., Rodriguez, V., Luna, M., McCredie, K. B., and Bodey, G. P. (1975): Successful control of systemic aspergillus niger infections in two patients with acute leukemia. *Cancer 36:2271–2276.*

Ghossein N. A., Bosworth, J. L., and Bases, R. E. (1975): The effect of radical radiotherpy on delayed hypersensitivity and the inflammatory response. *Cancer 35:1616–1620.*

Ghossein, N. A., Bosworth, J. L., Stacey, P., Muggia, F. M., and Rishnaswamy, V. (1975): Radiation related eosinophilia. Correlation with delayed hypersensitivity, lymphocyte count, and survival in patients treated by curative radiotherapy. *Radiology 117:413–417.*

Gleason, T. H., and Hamlin, W. B. (1974): Disseminated toxoplasmosis in the compromised host. *Arch Intern Med 134:1059–1062.*

Goffinet, D. R., Gratstein, E. J., and Merigan, T. C. (1972): Herpes zoster-varicella infections and lymphoma. *Ann Intern Med 76:235–240.*

Golde, D. W., and Cline, M. J. (1974): Regulation of granulopoiesis. *N Engl J Med 291:1388–1395.*

Goldman, J. M., and Aisenberg, A. C. (1970): Incidence of antibody to E B virus, herpes simplex, and cytomegalovirus in Hodgkin's disease. *Cancer 26:327–331.*

Goldman, J. M., and Lowenthal, R. M. (1975): *Leucocytes: Separation, Collection and Transfusion.* Academic Press, London.

Golub, S. H., O'Connell, T. X., and Morton, D. L. (1974): Correlation of in vivo and in vitro assays of immunocompetence in cancer patients. *Cancer Res 34:1833–1837.*

Gongaware, R. D., and Slanetz, C. A., Jr. (1973): Hartmann procedure for carcinoma of the sigmoid and rectum. *Ann Surg 178:28–30.*

Gontzea, I. (1974): *Nutrition and Anti-infectious Defence.* Karger, Basel.

Goodell, B., Jacobs, J. B., Powell, R. D., and DeVita, V. T. (1970): Pneumocystis carinii: The spectrum of diffuse interstitial pneumonia in patients with neoplastic diseases. *Ann Intern Med 72:337–340.*

Graham-Pole, J., Willoughby, M. L. N., Aitken, S., and Ferguson, A. (1975): Immune status of children with and without severe infection during remission of malignant disease. *Br Med J 2:467–470.*

Grange, M. J., Weisgerber, C., Montserrat, E., Teillet, F., and Reviron, J. (1975): Maladie de Hodgkin et entigène Australie. *Actual Hematol 9:111–120.*

Graw, R. G., Jr., Herzig, G. P., Perry, S., and Henderson, E. S. (1972): Normal granulocyte transfusion therapy. Treatment of septicemia due to gram-negative bacteria. *N Engl J Med 287:367–371.*

Greenman, R. L., Goodall, P. T., and King, D. (1975): Lung biopsy in immunocompromised host. *Am J Med 59:488–496.*

Gregory, L., Williams, R., and Thompson, E. (1972): Leucocyte function in Down's syndrome and acute leukaemia. *Lancet 1:1359–1361.*

Gremmel, H., and Schulte-Brinkmann, W. (1966): Besteht ein Kausalzusammenhang zwischen Strahlentherapie und Herpes Zoster. *Strahlentherapie 130:57–72.*

Griève, N. W. T. (1964): Monilial oesophagitis. *Br J Radiol 37:551–554.*

Grillo-Lopez, A. J., Rivera, E., Castillo-Staab, M., and Maldonado, N. (1971): Disseminated M. Kansasii infection in a patient with chronic granulocytic leukemia. *Cancer 28:476–481.*

Gröschel, D., Burgess, M. A., and Bodey, G. P. (1976): Gas gangrene like infection with *Bacillus cereus* in a lymphoma patient. *Cancer 37:988–991.*

Grose, W. E., Bodey, G. P., and Rodriguez, V. (1977): Sulfamethoxazole Trimethoprim for infections in cancer patients. *J Am Med Assoc 237:352–354.*

Gross, L., Manfredi, O. L., and Protos, A. A. (1973): Effect of cobalt-60 irradiation upon cell-mediated immunity. *Radiology 105:653–655.*

Haghbin, M., Armstrong, D., and Murphy, M. L. (1973): Controlled prospective trial of Pseudomonas aeruginosa vaccine in children with acute leukemia. *Cancer 32:761–766.*

Han, T., and Takita, H. (1972): Immunologic impairment in bronchogenic carcinoma: A study of lymphocyte response to phytohemagglutinin. *Cancer 30:616–620.*

Hancock, B. W., Bruce, L., Ward, A. M., and Richmond, J. (1976): Changes in immune status in patients undergoing splenectomy for the staging of Hodgkin's disease. *Br Med J 1:313–315.*

Hande, K. R., Witebsky, F. G., Brown, M. S., Schulman, C. B., Anderson, S. E., Jr., Levine, A. S., McLowry, J. D., and Chabner, B. A. (1976): Sepsis with a new species of *Corynebacterium. Ann Intern Med 85:423–426.*

Harris, J., Alexanian, R., Hersh, E. M., and Leary, W. (1969): Hodgkin's disease complicated by infection with mycobacterium kansasii. *Canad Med Assoc J 101:231–234.*

Harris, M. N., Gumport, S. L., Berman, I. R., and Bernard, R. W. (1973): Ilioinguinal lymph node dissection for melanoma. *Surg Gynecol Obstet 136:33–39.*

Hattori, A., Ihara, T., Iwasa, T., Kamiyo, H., Sakurai, M., Izawa, T., and Takahashi, M. (1976): Use of live varicella vaccine in children with acute leukaemia or other malignancies. *Lancet 2:210.*

Hefferman, A. G. A., and Asper, S. P., Jr. (1966): Insidious fungal disease. A clinicopathological study of secondary aspergillosis. *Bull Johns Hopkins Hosp 118:10–26.*

Heine, K. M. (1965): Zoster bei Leukose und Lymphogranulomatose. *Münch Med Wschr 107:1038–1041.*

Heineman, H. S., and Breen, F. A. (1975): Herpes simplex encephalitis in Hodgkin's disease. Isolation of drug-sensitive virus from brain following unsuccessful treatment with idoxuridine. *Cancer 36:1344–1347.*

Hendry, W. S., and Patrick, R. L. (1962): Observations on thirteen cases of pneumocystis carinii pneumonia. Am J Clin Pathol 38:401–405.

Henkel, J. S., Armstrong, D., Blevins, A., and Moody, M. D. (1970): Group A β-hemolytic Streptococcus bacteremia in a cancer hospital. J Am Med Assoc 211:983–986.

Hersh, E. M., Bodey, G. P., Nies, B. A., and Freireich, E. J. (1965): The causes of death in acute leukemia. A study of 414 patients from 1954–1963. J Am Med Assoc 193:105–109.

Herzig, R. H., Herzig, G. P., Graw, R. G., Bull, M. I., and Ray, K. K. (1977): Successful granulocyte transfusion therapy for gram-negative septicemia. A prospectively randomized controlled study. N Engl J Med 296:701–705.

Hesse, J., Andersen, E., Levine, P. H., Ebbesen, P., Halberg, P., and Reisher, J. I. (1973): Antibodies to Epstein-Barr virus and cellular immunity in Hodgkin's disease and chronic lymphatic leukemia. Int J Cancer 11:237–243.

Higby, D. J., Yates, J. W., Henderson, E. S., and Holland, J. F. (1975): Filtration leukapheresis for granulocyte transfusion therapy. Clinical and laboratory studies. N Engl J Med 292:761–766.

Hirshaut, Y., Gladc, P., Vieira, L. O. B. D., Aimbender, E., Dvorak, B., and Siltzbach, L. E. (1970): Saroidosis, another disease associated with serologic evidence for herpes-like virus infection. N Engl J Med 283:502–506.

Hirshaut, Y., Reagan, R. L., Perry, S., DeVita, V., Jr., and Barile, M. F. (1974): The search for a viral agent in Hodgkin's disease. Cancer 34:1080–1089.

Hoeprich, P. D., and Huston, A. C. (1975): Susceptibility of Coccidioides immunitis, Candida albicans and Cryptococcus neoformans to amphotericin B, flucytosine and clotrimazole. J Infect Dis 132:133–141.

Hoerni, B. (1972): Les engrenages pathologiques. Nouv Presse Med 1:53–54.

Hoerni, B. (1974): Influence of radiation therapy on the immune status of cancer patients, in Proceedings of the XIII International Congress of Radiology, Madrid, 1973, Excerpta Medica, Amsterdam, vol. 1, pp. 630–632.

Hoerni, B., Aubertin, J., Simon, G., and Chauvergne, J. (1971): Problèmes diagnostiques posés par les complications infectieuses de la maladie de Hodgkin. Bordeaux Med 4:1021–1030.

Hoerni, B., Castéra, M., and Chauvergne, J. (1976): L'omnipraticien dans la surveillance et le traitement des cancéreux. Bordeaux Med 9:1219–1228.

Hoerni, B., Chauvergne, J., Hoerni-Simon, G., Durand, M., Brunet, R., and Lagarde, C. (1976): BCG in the immunotherapy of Hodgkin's disease and non-Hodgkin's lymphomas. Results of a controlled trial including 60 patients. Cancer Immunol Immunother 1:109–112.

Hoerni, B., Chauvergne, J., and Parsi, M. (1970): La fièvre de la maladie de Hodgkin. Hypothèse pathogénique. Presse Med 78:1317–1319.

Hoerni, B., Hoerni-Simon, G., Durand, M., and Leleu, J. P. (1973): Maladie de Hodgkin chez un adulte insuffisant immunitaire. Bordeaux Med 6:1699–1703.

Hoerni, B., and Laporte, G. (1970). Immunological disorders in the aetiology of lymphoreticular neoplasms. Rev Eur Et Clin Biol 15:841–850.

Hoerni, B., Simon, G., and Chauvergne, J. (1972): Infections à herpes-virus au cours de la maladie de Hodgkin. Bordeaux Med. 5:771–778.

Hoerni, B., Vallat, M., Durand, M., and Pesme, D. (1977): Ocular toxoplasmosis and Hodgkin's disease. Report of two cases. Arch Ophtalmol, in press.

Hoerni, B., Vital, C., and Bonnaud, E. (1972): Leucémie aiguë lymphoblastique chez un sujet atteint d'ataxie-télangiecstasie. Acta Haematol 47:250–254.

Hoerni-Simon, G., Chauvergne, J., Durand, M., Eghbali, H., and Hoerni, B. (1977). Chimiothérapie discontinue des cancers lymphoprolifératifs à croissance lente. *Bordeaux Med 10:549–551.*

Hoffbrand, B. I. (1964): Hodgkin's disease and hypogammaglobulinemia: A rare association. *Br Med J 1:1156–1158.*

Homberg, J. C., Cartron, J., Ropars, C., Cavaroc, M. and Salmon, C. (1971): Anomalies immunologiques observées au cours des leucémies lymphoïdes chroniques hyperlymphocytaires. *Nouv Rev Fr Hematol 11:476–483.*

Hoover, R., and Fraumeni, J. F., Jr. (1973): Risk of cancer in renal-transplant recipients. *Lancet 2:55–57.*

Hoster, H. A., Zanes, R. P., and Von Haam, E. (1949): Studies in Hodgkin's syndrome. IX The association of "viral" hepatitis and Hodgkin's disease. *Cancer Res 9:473–480.*

Howard, R. J., and Simmons, R. L. (1974): Acquired immunologic deficiences after trauma and surgical procedures. *Surg Gynecol Obstet 139:771–782.*

Hughes, W. T. (1971a): Fatal infections in childhood leukemia. *Am J Dis Child 122:283–287.*

Hughes, W. T. (1971b). Leukemia monitoring with fungal bone marrow cultures. *J Am Med Assoc 218:441–443.*

Hughes, W. T., Price, R. A., Kim, H. K., Coburn, T. B., Grigsby, D., and Feldman, S. (1973): *Pneumocystis carinii* pneumonitis in children with malignancies. *J Pediat 82:404–415.*

Hughes W. T., and Smith, D. R. (1973): Infection during induction of remission in acute lymphocytic leukemia. *Cancer 31:1008–1014.*

Hunt, P. S., and Trotter, S. (1976): Lymphocyte response after surgery and blood transfusion. *J Surg Res 21:57–61.*

Iannini, P. B., Claffey, T., and Quintiliani, R. (1974): Bacteremic *Pseudomonas* pneumonia. *J Am Med Assoc 230:558–561.*

Ihde, D. C., and Armstrong, D. (1973): Clinical spectrum of infection due to bacillus species. *Am J Med 55:839–845.*

Inagaki, J., Rodriguez, V., and Bodey, G. P. (1974): Causes of death in cancer patients. *Cancer 33:568–573.*

Israel, L. (1972): Infections au cours des chimiothérapies anticancéreuses. *Nouv Presse Med 1:273–275.*

Iyer, R., Ravindranath, Y., Kulkarni, R., Philippart, A., Reed, J. O., Brough, A. J., and Zuelzer, W. W. (1976): Bilateral interstitital pneumonia in acute lymphoblastic leukemia. *Am J Hematol 1:225–235.*

Jager, B. K., and Stamm, W. P. (1973): Brain abscesses caused by free-living amoeba probably of the genus Hartmannella in a patient with Hodgkin's disease. *Lancet 2:1343–1345.*

Janeway C. A., and Rosen, F. S. (1966): The gammaglobulins. IV. Therapeutic uses of gammaglobulin. *N Engl J Med 275:826–831.*

Jawetz, E. (1968): The use of combinations of antimicrobial drugs. *Ann Rev Pharmacol 8:151–170.*

Jay, S. J., Johanson, W. G., and Pierce, A. K. (1975): The radiographic resolution of *Streptococcus pneumoniae* pneumonia. *N Engl J Med 293:798–801.*

Johanson, W. G., Pierce, A. K., and Sanford, J. P. (1969): Changing pharyngeal bacterial flora of hospitalized patients: emergence of gram-negative bacilli. *N Engl J Med 281:1137–1140.*

Johanson, W. G., Pierce, A. K., Sanford, J. P., and Thomas, G. D. (1972): Nosocomial respiratory infections with gram-negative bacilli. *Ann Intern Med 77:701–706.*

Johansson, B., Klein, G., Henle, W., and Henle, G. (1970): Epstein-Barr virus (EBV); associated antibody patterns in malignant lymphoma and leukemia. I. Hodgkin's disease. *Int J Cancer 6:450–462.*

Johnson, A. J., Aronson, D. L., and Williams, W. J. (1972): Clinical use of plasma and plasma fractions, in *Hematology,* W. J. Williams, E. Beutler, A. J., Erslev, and R. W. Rundles (Eds.), McGraw-Hill, New York, pp. 1329–1353.

Johnson, H. D., and Johnson, W. W. (1970): Pneumocystis carinii pneumonia in children with cancer. Diagnosis and treatment. *J Am Med Assoc '214:1067–1073.*

Jones, S. E., Griffith, K., Dombrowsky, P., and Gaines, J. A. (1977). Immunodeficiency in patients with non-Hodgkin lymphomas. *Blood 49:335–344.*

Jorgensen, J. H., Carvajal, H. F., and Chipps, B. E. (1973): Rapid detection of gram-negative bacteriuria by use of the Limulus endotoxin assay. *Appl Microbiol 26:43–48.*

Juel-Jensen, B. E., and MacCallum, F. O. (1972): *Herpes Simplex Varicella and Zoster Clinical Manifestations and Treatment.* Heinemann, London.

Juel-Jensen, B. E., MacCallum, F. O., Mackenzie, A. M. R., and Pike, M. C. (1970): Treatment of zoster with idoxuridine in dimethyl sulfoxide: Results of two double-bind controlled trials. *Br Med J 4:776–779.*

Kagnoff, M. F., Armstrong, D., and Blevins, A. (1972): Bacteroides bacteremia. Experience in a hospital for neoplastic diseases. *Cancer 29:245–251.*

Kammer, R. B., and Utz, J. P. (1974): Aspergillus species endocarditis. The new face of a not so rare disease. *Am J Med 56:506–521.*

Kaplan, M. H., Armstrong, D., and Rosen, P. (1974): Tuberculosis complicating neoplastic disease. A review of 201 cases. *Cancer 33:850–858.*

Karchmer, A. W., and Hirsch, M. S. (1973): Cytosine-arabinoside versus virus or man? *N Engl J Med 289:912–913.*

Katz, M. E., and Cassileth, P. A. (1977): Disseminated candidiasis in a patient with acute leukemia. Successful treatment with miconazole. *J Am Med Assoc 237:1124–1125.*

Kaufman, L., and Blumer, S. (1968): Value and interpretation of serological tests for the diagnosis of crytococcosis. *Appl Microbiol 16:1907–1912.*

Keating, M. J., and Penington, D. G. (1973): Prophylaxis against septicemia in acute leukaemia: The use of oral framycetin. *Med J Austr 2:213–217.*

Kenis, Y., Dustin, P., Jr., and Peltzer, T. (1959): Un cas de maladie de Hodgkin avec syndrome hématologique et sérologique de mononucléose infectieuse. *Acta Haematol 20:329–333.*

Kennedy, B. J., Bornstein, R., Brunning, R. D., and Oines, D. (1970): Breast involvement in acute lymphatic leukemia. Daunorubicine-induced remission: Pneumocystis carinii pneumonia. *Cancer 25:693–696.*

Kernec, J., de Labarthe, B., Le Freche, J. N., Ramée, M. P., Cormier, M., and Danrigal, A. (1974): Le brossage bronchique distal. Evolution des techniques. Exploitation des prélèvements. Résultats. *Rev Cytol Clin 7:33–41.*

Kersey, J. H., Spector, B. D., and Good, R. A. (1973): Primary immunodeficiency diseases and cancer: The immunodeficiency-cancer registry. *Int J Cancer 12:333–347.*

Ketover, B. P., Young, S. L., and Armstrong, D. (1973): Septicemia due to Aeromonas hydrophila. Clinical and immunological aspect. *J Infect Dis 127:284–290.*

Khan, A., Hill, J. M., MacLellan, A., Loeb, E., Hill, N. O., and Thaxton, S. (1975): Improvement in delayed hypersensitivity in Hodgkin's disease with transfer factor: Lymphapheresis and cellular immune reactions of normal donors. *Cancer* 36:86–89.

Klastersky, J. (1971a): Sensitivity to antibiotics of gram negative pathogens isolated from hospitalised patients having disseminated malignant diseases. *Eur J Cancer* 7:411–417.

Klastersky, J. (1971b): Antibiothérapie des infections graves en milieu hospitalier. *Presse Med* 79:1795–1799.

Klastersky, J. (1971c). Prophylactic use of antimicrobial agents. *Rev Eur Et Clin Biol* 16:11–15.

Klastersky, J. (1972a): Les infections opportunistes à candida: Considérations sur leur prévention. *Nouv Presse Med* 1:39–41.

Klastersky, J. (1972b): Les combinations d'antibiotiques. *Nouv Presse Med* 1:2041–2044.

Klastersky, J. (1973): Effectiveness of the carbenicillin-cephalothin combination against gram negative bacilli. *Am J Med Sci* 265:45–53.

Klastersky, J. (1974): Incidence and management of infections occurring in malignant lymphomas, in *I linfomi maligni*, P. Bucalossi et al. (Eds.), Casa Ambrosiana, Milan, pp. 367–375.

Klastersky, J., Cappel, R., and Daneau, D. (1972a): Bacterial colonization and clinical superinfection during antibiotic treatment of infections in patients with cancer. *Rev Et Clin Biol* 17:299–320.

Klastersky, J., Cappel, R., and Daneau, D. (1972b): Clinical significance of in vitro synergism between antibiotics in gram negative infections. *Antimicrob Agents Chemother* 12:470–475.

Klastersky, J., Cappel, R., and Daneau, D. (1973): Therapy with carbenicillin and gentamicin for patients with cancer and severe infections caused by gram negative rods. *Cancer* 31:331–336.

Klastersky, J., Cappel, R., Debusscher, L., and Stilmant, M. (1971): Pneumonia caused by gram-negative bacilli in hospitalized patients presenting malignant diseases. *Eur J Cancer* 7:329–336.

Klastersky, J., Cappel, R., Swings, G., and Vandenborre, L. (1971): Bacteriological and clinical activity of the ampicillin/gentamicin and cephalothin/gentamicin combinations. *Am J Med Sci* 262:283–290.

Klastersky, J., Daneau, D., and Verhest, A. (1972): Causes of death in patients with cancer. *Eur J Cancer* 8:149–154.

Klastersky, J., Debusscher, L., Weerts, D., and Daneau, D. (1974): Use of oral antibiotics in protected units environment: Clinical effectiveness and role in the emergence of antibiotic-resistant strains. *Pathol Biol* 22:5–12.

Klastersky, J., Geuning, C., Mouaward, E., and Daneau, D. (1972): Endotracheal gentamicin in bronchial infections in patients with tracheostomy. *Chest* 61:117–120.

Klasersky, J., Henri, A., Hensgens, C., and Daneau, D. (1974): Gram negative infections in cancer. Study of empiric therapy comparing carbenicillin-cephalothin with and without gentamicin. *J Am Med Assoc* 287:45–48.

Klastersky, J., Henri, A., Hensgens C., Vandenborre, and Daneau, D. (1973): Antipseudomonal drugs: comparative study of gentamicin, sisomicin and tobramicin in vitro and in human volunteers. *Eur J Cancer* 9:641–648.

Klastersky, J., Hensgens, C., and Debusscher, L. (1975): Empiric therapy for cancer patients, comparative study of ticaricillin-tobramycin, ticarillin-cephalothin and cephalothin-tobramycin. *Antimicrob Agents Chemoth* 7:640–645.

Klock, J. C., and Oken, R. L., (1976): Febrile neutrophilic dermatosis in acute myelogenous leukemia. *Cancer* 37:922–927.

Knospe, W. H., Loeb, V., Jr., and Huguley, C. M., Jr. (1974): Bi-weekly chlorambucil treatment of chronic lymphocytic leukemia. *Cancer* 33:555–562.

Krick, J. A., and Remington, J. S.(1976): Opportunistic invasive fungal infections in patients with leukemia and lymphoma. *Clin Haematol* 5:249–310.

Krick, J. A., Stinson, E. B., and Remington, J. S. (1975): Nocardia infection in heart transplant patients. *Ann Intern Med* 82:18–26.

Kun, L. E., and Johnson, R. E. (1975): Hematologic and immunologic status in Hodgkin's disease 5 years after radical radiotherapy. *Cancer* 36:1812–1816.

Kwan-Chung, K. J., Young, R. C., and Orlando, M. (1975): Pulmonary mucormycosis caused by *Cuminghamella elegans* in a patient with chronic myelogenous leukemia. *Am J Clin Pathol* 64:544–548.

Lacoste, G., and Mandoul, R. (1971): Candidoses bronchiques au cours du traitement des cancers bronchiques et des bronchites chroniques. *Rev Tuberc Pneumol* 35:543–550.

Lacut, J. Y., Leng, B., Buy, E., Boget, J. C., and Aubertin, J. (1974): Fièvre, infection et cancer. Espérience de la clinique médicale et des maladies infectieuses (A propos de 526 dossiers). *Bordeaux Med* 7:1319–1330.

Lacut, J. Y., Jaubert, D., Hoerni, B., Leng, B., and Aubertin, J. (1974): Les méningites bactériennes au cours des hémopathies malignes. *Bordeaux Med* 7:1363–1383.

Lamb, D., Pilney, R., Kelly, D. W., and Good, R. A. (1962): A comparative study of the incidence of anergy in patients with carcinoma, leukemia, Hodgkin's disease and other lymphomas. *J. Immunol* 89:555–558.

Landau, J. W., Newcomer, V. D., and Schultz, J. (1963): Aspergillosis. Report of two instances in children associated with acute leukemia and review of the pertinent literature. *Mycopathologia* 20:177–224.

Lang, J. M. (1973). Etude de la compétence immunologique dans la maladie de Hodgkin. *Pathol Biol* 21:285–297.

Langenhuysen, M. M. A. C., Cazemier, T., Houwen, B., Brouwers, T. M., Halie, M. R., The, T. H., and Nieweg, H. O. (1974): Antibodies to Epstein-Barr virus, cytomegalovirus and Australia antigen in Hodgkin's disease. *Cancer* 34:262–267.

Lau, W. K., and Young, L. S. (1976): Trimethoprim-Sulfamethoxazole treatment of pneumocystis carinii pneumonia in adult. *N Engl J Med* 295:716–718.

Lau, W. K., Young, L. S., and Remington, J. S. (1976): Pneumocystis carinii pneumonia. Diagnosis by examination of pulmonary secretions. *J Am Med Assoc* 236:2399–2402.

Laval, P., Besson, J., Meyer, G., Kleisbauer, J. P., Cesarini, J. P., and Rouquette, D. (1971): Surveillance des défenses immunitaires au cours du traitement des carcinomes bronchiques primitifs. *Bull Cancer* 58:91–102.

Lawton R. L., and Keehn, R. J. (1972): Bronchogenic cancer, sepsis and survival. *J Surg Oncol* 4:466–469.

Leclair, R. (1969): Descriptive epidemiology of interstitial pneumocystic pneumonia: An analysis of 107 cases from the United States, 1955–1967. *Am Rev Resp Dis* 99:542–547.

Lee, Y. T. N. (1977): Peripheral lymphocyte count and subpopulations of T and B lymphocytes in benign and malignant diseases. *Surg Gynecol Obstet* 144:435–450.

Legendre, P., Merlet, M., Lacut, J. Y., Leng, B., and Aubertin, J. (1976): Du test au NBT dans de diagnostic d'une infection bactérienne. *Bordeaux Med* 9:1619–1624.

Lehane, D. E., and Lane, M. (1974): Immunocompetence in advanced cancer patients prior to chemotherapy. *Oncology 30:458–466.*

Lehrer, R. I., and Cline, M. J. (1971): Leukocyte candidacidal activity and resistance to systemic candidiasis in patient wth cancer. *Cancer 27:1211–1217.*

Leigh, D. A. (1974): Clinical importance of infections due to Bacteroides fragilis and role in antibiotic therapy. *Br Med J 3:225–228.*

Lemaire, A., Debray, J., Blanchon, P., and You Kim Yean (1965): Aspects ganglionnaires et sanguins de la toxoplasmose acquise de l'adulte (A propos de 14 observations personnelles). *Bull Mem Soc Med Hop Paris 116:335–351.*

Leng, B., Lacut, J. Y., Renou, J., and Aubertin, J. (1974): Les cryptococcoses neuro-méningées. Etude clinique et thérapeutique. *Bordeaux Med 7:1385–1394.*

Leng-Levy, J., Aubertin, J., Leng, B., Lacut, J. Y., and Le Gall, F. (1971); Signification de la fièvre chez les cancéreux. *Maroc Med 51:502–510.*

Leng-Levy, J., David-Chaussé, J., and Gibaud, H. (1961): Septicémies au cours des néoplasmes. *J Med Bordeaux 138:1318–1323.*

Lerner, P., Wolinsky, E., Gavan, T., McHenry, M., Rosenthal, M., Gopalakrishna, K. V., and Tan, J. S. (1975): Group B streptococcal bacteremia in adults. Program and abstracts of XVth Interscience Conference on antimicrobial agents and chemotherapy, 24–26 September, 1975, Washington, D.C. Abstract No. 44.

Le Treut, A., Hoerni, B., Durand, M., and Lagarde, C. (1972): Les réactions fébriles post-lymphographiques dans les réticulopathies malignes. *J Radiol Electrol 53:143–149.*

Le Treut, A., Lagarde, C., Stoll, R., Meugé, C., and Bruzat, M. H. (1971): Le poumon après lymphographie. *J Radiol Electrol 52:317–325.*

Levi, J. A., Vincent, P. C., and Jennis, F. (1973): Prophylactic oral antibiotics in the management of acute leukemia. *Med J Austr 1:1025–1029.*

Levin, A. G., Miller, D. G., and Southam, C. M. (1968): Lymphocyte transfer tests in cancer patients and healthy people. *Cancer 22:500–506.*

Levine, A. S., Graw, R. G., Jr., and Young, R. C. (1972): Management of infections in patients with leukemia and lymphoma. Current concepts and experimental approaches. *Semin Hematol 9:141–179.*

Levine, A. S., Siegel, S. E., Schreiber, A. D., Hauser, J., Preisler, H., Goldtein, I. M., Seidler, F., Simon, R., Perry, S., Bennett, J. E., and Henderson, E. S. (1973): Protected environments and prophylactic antibiotics. A prospective controlled study of their utility in the therapy of acute leukemia. *N Engl J Med 288:477–483.*

Levine, P. H., Ablashi, D. V., Berard, C. W., Carbone, P. P., Waggoner, D. E., and Malan, L. (1971): Elevated antibody titers to Epstein-Barr virus in Hodgkin's disease. *Cancer 27:416–421.*

Levine P. H., Merrill, D. A., Bethlenfalvay, N. C., Dabich, L., Stevens, D. A., and Waggoner, D. E. (1971): A longitudinal comparison of antibodies to Epstein-Barr virus and clinical parameters in chronic lymphocytic leukemia and chronic myelocytic leukemia. *Blood 38:479–484.*

Levitan, A. A., and Perry, S. (1968): The use of an isolater system in cancer chemotherapy. *Am J Med 44:234–242.*

Levy, M. A., Senior, R. M., and Sneider, R. E. (1974): Severe thrombocytopenic purpura complicating pentamidine therapy for Pneumocystis carinii pneumonia. *Cancer 34:441–443.*

Lewis, J. L., and Rabinovich, S. (1972): The wide spectrum of cryptococcal infections. *Am J Med 53:315–322.*

Liabeuf, A., Kourilsky, F. M. (1975): Système antigénique de la tumeur de Burkitt et le virus d'Epstein-Barr. *Actual Hematol 9:228–242.*

Lightdale, C. J., Wolf, D. J., Marcucci, R. A., and Salyer, W. R. (1977): Herpetic esophagitis in patients with cancer: ante mortem diagnosis by brush cytology. *Cancer 39:223–226.*

Littenberg, R. L., Taketa, R. M., Alazraki, N. P., Halpern, S. E., and Ashburn, W. L. (1973): Gallium-67 for localizations of septic lesions. *Ann Intern Med 79:403–406.*

Loiseau-Marolleau, M. L. (1970a): Contribution à l'étude de l'infection aucours des leucémies aiguës. (Etude de 139 cas.) Les paramètres de l'infection: neutropénie et immunodépression. Rôle respectif de la flore endogène et des contaminations exogènes. *Pathol Biol 18:975–983.*

Loiseau-Marolleau, M. L. (1970b): Contribution à l'étude de l'infection au cours des leucémies aiguës. (Etude de 139 cas.) II Signification des hémocultures positives. *Pathol Biol 18:1089–1096.*

Lorber, B., and Swenson, R. M. (1974): Bacteriology of aspiration pneumonia. A prospective study of community and hospital-acquired cases. *Ann Intern Med 81:329–331.*

Louria, D. B., Hensle, T., Armstrong, D., Collins, H. S., Blevins, A., Krugman, D., and Buse, M. (1967): Listeriosis complicating malignant disease. A new association. *Ann Intern Med 67:261–281.*

Louria, D. B., Steff, D. P., and Bennett, B. (1962): Disseminated moniliasis in the adult. *Medicine 41:307–337.*

Lowenthal, R. M., Grossman, L., Goldman, J. M., Storring, R. A., Buskard, N. A., Park, D. S., Murphy, N. A., and Spiers, A. S. D. (1975): Granulocyte transfusions in treatment of infections in patients with acute leukaemia and aplastic anaemia. *Lancet 1:353–358.*

Luft, F. C., Rissing, J. P., White, A., and Brooks, G. F., (1976): Infections or neoplasms as causes of prolonged fever in cancer patients. *Am J Med Sci 272:65–74.*

Luna, A. M., and Lichtiger, B. (1971): Disseminated toxoplasmosis and cytomegalovirus infection complicating Hodgkin's disease. *Am J Clin Path 55:499–505.*

Lunde, M. N., Gelderman, A. H., Hayes, S. L., and Vogel, C. L. (1970): Serologic diagnosis of active toxoplasmosis complicating malignant diseases. Usefulness of IgM antibodies and gel-diffusion. *Cancer 25:637–643.*

Lundy, J., Raaf, J. H., Deakins, S., Wanebo, H. J., Jacobs, D. A., Lee, T. D., Jacobowitz, D., Spear, C., and Oettgen, H. F. (1975): The acute and chronic effects of alcohol on the human immune system. *Surg Gynecol Obstet 141:212–218.*

Lynfield, Y. L., Farhangi, M., and Runnels, J. L. (1969): Generalized herpes simplex complicating lymphoma. *J Am Med Assoc 207:944–945.*

Mandel, M. A., Dvorak, K., and Decosse, J. J. (1973): Salivary immunoglobulins in patients with oropharyngeal and bronchopulmonary carcinoma. *Cancer 31:1408–1413.*

Manes, J. L., and Blair, O. M. (1976): Disseminated *Mycobacterium kansasii* infection complicating hairy cell leukemia. *J Am Med Assoc 236:1878–1879.*

Marée, D. (1968): La chimiothérapie par infusions intra-artérielles (A propos de 210 traitements en cancérologie cervicofaciale). Thèse, Bordeaux, No. 121.

Marsh, J. C., and Von Graevenitz, A. (1973): Recurrent Corynebacterium equi infection with lymphoma. *Cancer 32:147–149.*

Marty, A. T., Miyamoto, A. M., and Philips, P. A. (1975): Definitive diagnosis of pulmonary lesions in leukemia and lymphoma. *Arch Surg 110:1199–1202.*

Massey, F. C., Lane, L. L., and Imbriglia, J. E. (1953): Acute infectious mononucleosis and Hodgkin's disease occurring simultaneously in same patient. *J Am Med Assoc 151:994–997.*

Masson, R., Fière, D., Lahnèche, B., Cordat, C., Berger, F., and Revol, L. (1975): Toxoplasmose encephalique pseudo-tumorale au cours d'une hémopathie. Deux observations. *Nouv Presse Med 4:2499–2502.*

Masur, H., Hook, E., and Armstrong, D., (1976): A *Trichomonas* species in a mixed microbial meningitis. *J Am Med Assoc 236:1978–1979.*

Mathé, G., Schwarzenberg, L., Hayat, M., and Schneider, M. (1969): Chimiothérapie de la leuémie L1210: Comparaison, pour 7 composées, des effets de l'administration continue sur 20 jours et de l'administration d'une dose unique, massive, précoce ou tardive. *Rev Fr Et Clin Biol 13:951–960.*

Maupas, P., Werner, B., Larouzé, B., Millman, I., London, W. T., O'Connell, A. Blumberg, B. S., Saimot, G., Payet, M. (1975): Antibody to hepatitis-B core antigen in patients with primary hepatic carcinoma. *Lancet 2:9–11.*

McBride, M. E., Duncan, C., Bodey, G. P., and McBride, C. M. (1976): Microbial skin flora of selected cancer patients and hospital personnel. *J Clin Microbiol 3:14–20.*

McKelvey, E. M., and Kwaan, H. C. (1969): Cytosine arabinoside therapy for disseminated herpes zoster in a patient with IgG pyroglobulinemia. *Blood 34:706–711.*

McKneally, M. F., Maver, C., and Kausel, H. W. (1976): Regional immunotherapy of lung cancer with intrapleural B.C.G. *Lancet 1:377–379.*

Medoff, G., and Kobayashi, G. S. (1972): Pulmonary mucormycosis. *N Engl J Med 286:86–87.*

Melnick, J. L., and Rawls, W. E. (1974): The causative role of herpesvirus type 2 in cervical cancer. *Cancer 34:1375–1385.*

Metcalfe, D., and Hughes, W. T. (1972): Effects of methotrexate on group A beta hemolytic streptococci and streptococcal infection. *Cancer 30:588–593.*

Meyer, R. D., Kaplan, M. H., Ong, M. O., and Armstrong, D. (1973): Cutaneous lesions in disseminated mucormycosis. *J Am Med Assoc 225:737–738.*

Meyer, R. D., Lewis, R. P., Carmalt, E. D., and Finegold, S. M. (1975): Amikacin therapy for serious Gram negative bacillary infections. *Ann Int Med 83:790–800.*

Meyer, R. D., Young, L. S., Armstrong, D., and Yu, B. (1973): Aspergillosis complicating neoplastic disease. *Am J Med 54:6–15.*

Meyers, B. R., Hirschman, S. Z., and Axelrod, J. A. (1972): Current patterns of infection in multiple myeloma. *Am J Med 52:87–92.*

Middleman, E. L., Watanabe, A., Kaiser, H., and Bodey, G. P. (1972): Antibiotic combinations for infections in neutropenic patients. Evaluation of carbenicillin plus either cephalothin or kanamycin. *Cancer 30:573–579.*

Miller, D. G. (1968): The immunologic capability of patients with lymphomas. *Cancer Res 28:1441–1448.*

Miller, M. E. (1975): Pathology of chemotaxis and random mobility. *Sem Hematol 12:59–82.*

Mirsky, H. S., and Cuttner, J. (1972): Fungal infection in acute leukemia. *Cancer 30:348–352.*

Mitus, A., Holloway, A., Evans, A. E., and Enders, J. F. (1962): Attenuated measles vaccine in children with acute leukemia. *Am J Dis Child 103:413–418.*

Molander, D. W., and Pack, G. T. (1968): *Hodgkin's Disease.* Thomas, Springfield, Ill.

Mollaret, H. H., Omland, T., Henriksen, S. D., Baeroe, P. R., Rykner, G., and Scavizzi, M. (1971): Les septicémies humaines à "Yersinia enterocolitica." A propos de 17 cas récents. *Presse Med* 79:345–348.

Monfardini, S., Gee, T., Fred, J., and Clarkson, B. (1973): Survival in chronic myelogenous leukemia: influence of treatment and extent of disease at diagnosis. *Cancer* 31:492–501.

Montgomerie, J. Z., Edwards, J. E., Jr., and Guze, L. B. (1975): Synergism of amphotericin B and 5-fluorocytosine for candida species. *J Infect Dis* 132:82–86.

Moore, D. M., Cheuk, S. F., Morton, J. D., Berlin, R. D., and Wood, W. B. (1970): Studies on the pathogenesis of fever. XVIII. Activation of leukocytes for pyrogen production. *J Exp Med* 131:179–188.

Mordasini, R. C., Keller, H., Schlumpf, E., and Riva, G. (1972): Humorale Infektabwehrschwäche bei paraproteinämischen Erkrankungen. *Schweiz Med Wschr* 102:625–635.

Moulinier, B., Lambert, R., Grenier-Boley, P., and Brumière, J. (1972): Les mycoses de l'oesophage. *Nouv Presse Med* 1:2629 2632.

Muller, S. A. (1967): Association of zoster and malignant disorders in children. *Arch Derm Chicago* 96:657–664.

Muller, S. A., Herrmann, E. C., Jr., and Winkelmann, R. K. (1972): Herpes simplex infections in hematologic malignancies. *Am J Med* 50:102–114.

Nachum, R., Lipsey, A., and Siegel, S. E. (1973): Rapid detection of gram-negative bacterial meningitis by the limulus lysate test. *N Engl J Med* 289:931–934.

Nagel, G. A. (1971): Immunosuppression: ein paraneoplastisches Syndrome. *Schweiz Med Wschr* 101:470–474.

Naito, H., Toya, S., Shizawa, H., Iizaka, Y., and Tsukumo, D. (1973): High incidence of acute post operative meningitis and septicemia in patients undergoing craniotomy with ventriculoatrial shunt. *Surg Gynecol Obstet* 137:810–812.

Nakashima, T., Okuda, K., Kajiro, M., Sakamoto, K., Kubo, Y., and Shimokawa, Y. (1975): Primary liver cancer coincident with Schistomiasis japonica. A study of 24 necropsies. *Cancer* 36:1483–1489.

Narayan, O., Penney, J. B., Jr., Johnson, R. T., Herndon, R. M., and Weiner, L. P. (1973): Etiology of progressive multifocal leukoencephalopathy. Identification of Papovavirus. *N Engl J Med* 289:1278–1282.

Nathorst-Windahl, G., Hesselman, B. H., Sjöström, B., and Ponten, J. (1964): Massive fatal pneumocystis pneumonia in leukemia. Report of two cases. *Acta Pathol Microbiol Scand* 62:472–480.

Nauta, E. M., and Van Furth, R. (1975): Infection. in immunodepressed patients. *Infection* 3:202–208.

Neary, M. P., Allen, J., Okubadejo, O. A., and Payne, J. H. (1973): Preoperative vaginal bacteria and postoperative infections in gynaecological patients. *Lancet* 2:1291–1294.

Neiman, P. E., Thomas, E. D., Reeves, W. C., Ray, C. G., Sale, G., Lerner, K. G., Buckner, C. D., Clift, R. A., Storb, R., Weiden, P. L., and Fefer, A. (1974): Opportunistic infection and interstitital pneumonia following marrow transplantation for aplastic anemia and hematologic malignancy. *Transplant Proc* 8:663–667.

Neu, H. C. (1971): Toxoplasmose, complication des affections malignes. *Rev Med Paris* 12:487–490.

Nixon, D. W., and Aisenberg, A. C. (1972): Fatal Hemophilus influenzae in an asymptomatic splenectomized Hodgkin's disease patient. *Ann Intern Med* 77:69–71.

Northey, D., Adess, M. L., Hartsuck, J. M., and Rhoades, E. R. (1974): Microbial surveillance in a surgical intensive care unit. *Surg Gynecol Obstet* 139:321–325.

Nowoslawski, A., Brozosko, W. J., Madalinski, K., and Krawczynski, K. (1970): Cellular localization of Australia antigen in the liver of patients with lymphoproliferative disorders. *Lancet* 1:494–498.

Oberling, F., Giron, C., Bareiss, M. O., Lang, J. M., Reeb, E., Goetz, M. L., and Lavillaureix, J. (1975): Vaccinations anti-pyocyaniques et anti-staphylococciques au cours d'hémopathies malignes. *Nouv Rev Fr Hematol* 15:386–390.

O'Carroll, D. I., McKenna, R. W., and Brunning, R. D. (1976): Bone marrow manifestations of Hodgkin's disease. *Cancer* 38:1717–1728.

O.E.R.T.C. Groupe coopérateur Leucémies et Hématosarcomes (1975): Unité de soins intesifs hématocancérologiques. Leur rôle dans l'efficacité des chimiothérapies cytostatiques. *Nouv Presse Med* 4:1553–1556.

Okubadejo, O. A., Green, P. J., and Payne, D. J. H. (1973): Bacteroides infection among hospital patients. *Br Med J* 2:212–214.

Orita, K., Miwa, H., Fukada, H., Yumura, M., Uchida, Y., Mamnami, T. Konaga, E., and Tanaka, S. (1976): Preoperative cell-mediated immune status of gastric cancer patients. *Cancer* 38:2343–2348.

Oster, M. W., Gelrud, L. G., Lotz, M. J., Herzig, G. P., and Johnston, G. S. (1975): Psoas abscess localization by gallium scan in aplastic anemia. *J Am Med Assoc* 232:377–379.

Padgett, B. L., Walker, D. L., Zurhein, G. M., Eckroade, R. J., Dessel, B. H. (1971): Cultivation of papova-like virus from human brain with progressive multifocal leucoencephalopathy. *Lancet* 1:1257–1260.

Parry, M. F., and Neu, H. C. (1976): Ticarcillin for treatment of serious infections with Gram-negative bacteria. *J Infect Dis* 134:476–485.

Pennington, J. E. (1976): Successful treatment of Aspergillus pneumonia in hematologic neoplasia. *N Engl J Med* 295:426–427.

Pennington, J. E., Gibbons, N. D., Strobeck, J. E., Simpson, G. L., and Myerowitz, R. L. (1976): Bacillus species infection in patients with hematologic neoplasia. *J Am Med Assoc* 235:1473–1474.

Pennington, J. E., Reynolds, H. Y., and Carbone, P. (1973): Pseudomonas pneumonia. A retrospective study of 36 cases. *Am J Med* 55:155–160.

Pennington, J. E., Reynolds, H. Y., Wood, R. E., Robinson, R. A., and Levine, A. S. (1975): Use of a Pseudomonas aeruginosa vaccine in patients with acute leukemia and cystic fibrosis. *Am J Med* 58:629–636.

Perera, D. R., Western, K. A., Johnson, H. D., Johnson, W. W., Schultz, M. G., and Akers, P. V. (1970): Pneumocystis carinii pneumonia in a hospital for children. Epidemiologic aspects. *J Am Med Assoc* 214:1074–1078.

Pickering, L. K., Anderson, D. C., Choi, S., and Feigin, R. D. (1975): Leukocyte function in children with malignancies. *Cancer* 35:1365–1371.

Pierce, L. E., and Jenkins, R. B. (1973): Herpes zoster ophthalmicus treated with cytarabine. *Arch Ophthalmol Chicago* 89:21–24.

Plager, J. E. (1976): Association of renal injury with combined cephalothin-gentamicin therapy among patients severely ill with malignant disease. *Cancer* 37:1937–1943.

Plesnicar, S. (1972): Immunoglobulins in carcinoma of the uterine cervix. *Acta Radiol Ther* 11:37–47.

Pollak, A. A., Berger, S. A., Richmond, S. A., Simberkoff, M. S., and Rahal, J. J. (1977): Amikacin therapy for serious Gram-negative infections. *J Am Med Assoc 237:562–564.*

Preisler, H. D., Goldstein, I. M., and Henderson, E. S. (1970): Gastrointestinal "sterilization" in the treatment of patients with acute leukemia. *Cancer 26:1076–1081.*

Preisler, H. D., Hasenclever, H. F., and Henderson, E. S. (1971): *Anti-Candida* antibodies in patients with acute leukemia: Prospective study. *Am J Med 51:352–361.*

Pruzanski, W., Leers, W. D., and Wardlaw, A. C. (1973): Bacteriolytic and bactericidal activity in monocytic and myelomonocytic leukemia with hyperlysozymemia. *Cancer Res 33:867–873.*

Pruzanski, W., and Saito, S. (1974). Influence of chemotherapeutic agents on the antibacterial activity of normal and leukemic sera. *J Natl Cancer Inst 52:643–647.*

Prystonsky, S. D., Vogelstein, B., Ettinger, D. S., Merz, W. G., Kaiser, H., Sulica, V. I., and Zinkham, W. H. (1976): Invasive aspergillosis. *N Engl J Med 295:655–658.*

Pujet, P. P., Raphael, M., Devergie, A., Chomette, G., and Binet, J. L. (1974). Pneumopathie à pneumocystis carinii compliquant une sarcomatose ganglionnaire de type plasmocytaire. *Ann Med Interne 125:261–266.*

Pullan, C. R., Noble, T. C., Scott, D. J., Wisniewski, K., and Gardner, P. S. (1976): Atypical measles infections in leukaemic children on immunosuppressive treatment. *Br Med J 1:1562–1565.*

Purtillo, D. T., Meyers, W. M., and Connor, D. H. (1974): Fatal strongyloidiasis in immunosuppressed patients. *Am J Med 56:488–493.*

Putman, C. E., Curtis, A. M., Simeone, J. F., and Jensen, P. (1975): *Mycoplasma* pneumonia. Clinical and roentgenographic patterns. *Am J Roentgen Radium Ther Nucl Med 124:417–422.*

Raben, M., Walach, N., Galili, U., and Schlesinger, M. (1976): The effect of radiation therapy on lymphocyte subpopulations in cancer patients. *Cancer 37:1417–1421.*

Ragab, A. H., Lindquist, K. J., Vietti, T. J., Choi, S. C., and Osterland, C. K. (1970): Immunoglobulin pattern in childhood leukemia. *Cancer 26:890–894.*

Ramsay, G. C., and Meyer, R. D. (1973): Cavitary fungus disease of the lungs. *Radiology 109:29–32.*

Rapin, M., Duval, J., Le Gall, J. R., Soussy, C. J., Lemaire, F., and Harari, A. (1975): Les septicémies de surinfection en réanimation. Leur prévention par la restriction de l'antibiothérapie. *Noux Presse Med 4:483–486.*

Rassiga-Pidot, A. L., and McIntyre, O. R. (1974): *In vitro* leukocyte interferon production in patients with Hodgkin's disease. *Cancer Res 34:2995–3002.*

Rivera, E., Maldonado, N., Velez-Garcia, D., Grillo, A. J., and Malaret, G. (1970): Hyperinfection syndrome with *Strongyloides stercoralis. Ann Intern Med 72:199–204.*

Rivera, R., and Cangir, A. (1975): *Trichosporon* sepsis and leukemia. *Cancer 36:1106–1110.*

Roberts, M. M., Bathgate, E. M., and Stevenson, A. (1975): Serum immunoglobulin levels in patients with breast cancer. *Cancer 36:221–224.*

Rodriguez, V., Burgess, M., and Bodey, G. P. (1973): Management of fever of unknown origin in patients with neoplasms and neutropenia. *Cancer 32:1007–1012.*

Rodriguez, V., Whitecar, J. P., and Bodey, G. P. (1969): Therapy of infections with the combination of carbenicillin and gentamicin. *Antimicrob Agents Chemother 9:386–390.*

Rogers, R. S., III, and Tindall, J. P. (1972): Herpes zoster in children. *Arch Derm Chicago 106:204–207.*

Rogers, W. A., Jr., and Nelson, B. (1966): Strongyloidiasis and malignant lymphoma. "Opportunistic infection" by a nematode. *J Am Med Assoc 195:685–687.*

Rosen, P., Armstrong, D., and Ramos, C. (1972): *Pneumocystis carinii* pneumonia: Clinicopathologic study of 20 patients with neoplastic diseases. *Am J Med 53:428–436.*

Rosen, P., and Hajdu, S. Cytomegalovirus inclusion disease at autopsy of patients with cancer. *Am J Clin Pathol 55:749–756.*

Rosenblum, W. I., and Hadfield, M. G. (1972): Granulomatous angitis of nervous system in cases of herpes zoster and lymphosarcoma. *Neurology (Minneap) 22:348–354.*

Rosenthal, S., and Tager, I. B. (1975): Prevalence of Gram-negative rods in the normal pharyngeal flora. *Ann Intern Med 83:355–357.*

Rosner, F., Gabriel, F. D., Taschdjian, C. L., Cuesta, M. B., and Kozinn, P. J. (1971): Serologic diagnosis of systemic candidiasis in patients with acute leukemia. *Am J Med 51:54–62.*

Roth, J. A., Siegel, S. E., Levine, A. S., and Berard, C. W. (1971): Fatal recurrent toxoplasmosis in patient initially infected via leukocyte transfusion. *Am J Clin Pathol 56:601–605.*

Roujeau, J., Galian, A., Ponchon, Y., Segrestaa, J. M., Caulin, C., Manicacci, M., and Dentan, M. (1971): Cryptococcose: maladie d'opportunité. *Sem Hop Paris 47:832–840.*

Ruck-deschel, J. C., Codish, S. D., Stranahan, A., and McKneally, M. F. (1972): Postoperative empyema improves survival in lung cancer. Documentation and analysis of a natural experiment. *N Engl J Med 287:1013–1017.*

Ruskin, J., and Remington, J. S. (1967): The compromise host and infection. I. Pneumocystis carinii pneumonia. *J Am Med Assoc 202:1070–1074.*

Sabath, L. D., and Abraham, E. P. (1964): Synergistic action of penicillin and cephalsporins against Pseudomonas pyocyanea. *Nature 204:1066–1069.*

Sadoff, L., and Goldsmith, O. (1971): False positive infectious mononucleosis spot test in pancreatic carcinoma. *J Am Med Assoc 218:1297–1298.*

Salmon, S. E. (1973): Immunoglobulin synthesis and tumor kinetics of multiple myeloma. *Semin Hematol 10:135–147.*

Salmon, S. E., Samal, B. A., Hayes, D. M., Hosley, H., Miller, S. P., and Schilling, A. (1967): Role of gammaglobulin for immunoprophylaxis in multiple myeloma. *N Engl J Med 277:1336–1340.*

Sarosi, G. A., Voth, D. W., Dahl, B. A., Doto, I. L., and Tosh, F. E. (1971): Disseminated histoplasmosis. Result of a long term follow-up. A center for disease control cooperative mycoses study. *Ann Intern Med 75:511–516.*

Sathmary, M. N. (1958): Bacillus subtilis septicemia and generalized aspergillosis in a patient with acute myeloblastic leukemia. *NY State J Med 58:1870–1876.*

Say, C. C., and Donegan, W. (1974): A biostatistical evaluation of complications from mastectomy. *Surg Gynecol Obstet 138:370–376.*

Schaefer, J. C., Yu, B., and Armstrong, D. (1976): An Aspergillus immunodiffusion test in the early diagnosis of aspergillosis in adult leukemia patients. *Am Rev Resp Dis 113:325–329.*

Schaison, G., Weisgerber, C., and Chavelet, F. (1971): Varicelle et leucémie. *Actual Hemat 5:112–122.*

Schellhammer, P. F., Bracken, R. B., Bean, M. A., Pinsky, C. M., and Whitmore,

W. F., Jr. (1976): Immune evaluation with skin testing. A study of testicular, prostate and bladder neoplasms. *Cancer 38:149–156.*

Schiffer, C. A., Buchholz, D. H., Aisner, J., Betts, S. W., and Wiernik, P. H. (1975): Clinical experience with transfusion of granulocytes obtained by continuous flow filtration leukopheresis. *Am J Med 58:373–381.*

Schimpff, S. C., Greene, W. H., Young, W. M., Fortner, C. L., Jepsen, L., Cusack, N., Block, J. B., and Wiernik, P. H. (1975): Infection prevention in acute non-lymphocytic antibiotic prophylaxis. *Ann Intern Med 82:351–358.*

Schimpff, S. C., Greene, W. H., Young, V. M., and Wiernik, P. H. (1973): *Pseudomonas* septicemia: Incidence, epidemiology, prevention and therapy in patients with advanced cancer. *Eur J Cancer 9:449–455.*

Schimpff, S. C., Greene, W. H., Young, V. M., and Wiernik, P. H. (1974): Significance of Pseudomonas aeruginosa in the patient with leukemia or lymphoma. *J Infect Dis 130 (suppl.): S24–S31.*

Schimpff, S. C., Landesman, S., Hahn, D. M., Standlford, H. C., Fortner, C. L., Young, V. M., and Wiernik, P. H. (1976): Ticarcillin in combination with cephalothin or gentimicin as empiric antibiotic therapy in granulocytopenic cancer patients. *Antimicrob Agents Chemother 10:837–844.*

Schimpff, S. C., O'Connel, M. J., Greene, W. H., and Wiernik, P. H. (1975): Infections in 92 splenectomized patients with Hodgkin's disease. A clinical review. *Am J Med 59:695–701.*

Schimpff, S. C., Satterlee, W., Young, V. M., and Serpick, A. (1971): Empiric therapy with carbenicillin and gentamicin for febrile patients with cancer and granulocytopenia. *N Engl J Med 284:1061–1065.*

Schimpff, S. C., Wiernik, P. H., and Block, J. B. (1972): Rectal abscesses in cancer patients. *Lancet 2:844–847.*

Schimpff, S. C., Young, V. M., Greene, W. H., Vermeulen, G. D., Moody, M. R., and Wiernik, P. H. (1972): Origin of infection in acute non-lymphocytic leukemia. Significance of hospital acquisition of potential pathogens. *Ann Intern Med 77:707–714.*

Schneider, M. (1968): Effet de chimiothérapies cytostatiques sur une réaction d'hypersensibilité retardée. *Rev Fr Et Clin Biol 13:877–880.*

Schneider, M., Schwarzenberg, L., Amiel, J. L., Cattan, A., Schlumberger, J. R., Hayat, M., deVassal, F., Jasmin, C., Rosenfeld, C., and Mathé, G. (1969): Pathogen-free isolation unit. Three years' experience. *Br Med J 1:836–839.*

Schrub, J., Bocquet, J. P., and Forthomme, J. (1967): Association de maladie de Hodgkin, cryptococcose et déficit en immunoglobuline (A propos d'une observation). *Arch Anat Pathol 15:14–24.*

Schwartz, S., Colvin, M., Himmelsback, D. K., and Frei, E. (1968): The effect of bacterial suppression and reverse isolation on intensive cancer chemotherapy. *Clin Res 13:48.*

Schwarzenberg, L., Cattan, A., Schneider, M., Schlumberger, J. R., Amiel, J. L., and Mathé, G. (1966): La "réanimation hématologique". II. Correction des désordres graves des leucocytes et des immunoglobulines. La greffe de moelle osseuse. *Presse Med 74:1061–1065.*

Schwarzenberg L., Mathé, G., Amiel, J. L., Cattan, A., Schneider, M., Schlumberger, J. R., (1966): Le traitement symptomatique de l'agranulocytose par les transfusions de globules blancs. *Presse Med 74:1057–1060.*

Sedaghatian, M. R., and Singer, D. B. (1972): Pneumocystis carinii in children with malignant disease. *Cancer 29:772–777.*

Sedgwick, R. P., Boder, E. (1972): Ataxia-telagniectasia. In *Handbook of Clinical Neurology*, P. J. Vinken, and G. W. Bryn, (Eds.), North-Holland, Amsterdam, Vol. 14, chap. 10, pp. 267–339.

Sehdev, M. K., Dowling, M. D., Seal, S. H., and Stearns, M. W. (1973): Perianal and anorectal complications in leukemia. *Cancer 31:149–152.*

Selz, B., and Novotny, Z. (1976): Klinisches Bild des Cryptococcus-neoformans Infektion. *Schweiz Med Wschr 106:1238–1242.*

Senn, H. J., and Jungi, W. F. (1975): Neutrophil migration in health and disease. *Sem Hematol 12:27–45.*

Senn, H. J., Rhomberg, W. U., and Jungi, W. F. (1971:) Störung der leukozytären Abwehrfunktion als paraneoplastischer Syndrom bei Hämoblastosen. *Schweiz Med Wschr 101:466–469.*

Shadony, S., Wagner, G., Espinel-Ingroff, A., and Davis, B. A. (1975): In vitro studies with combinations of 5-fluorocytosine and amphotericin B. *Antimicrob Agents Chemother 8:117–121.*

Shanbrom, E., Miller, S., and Haar, H. (1960): Herpes zoster in hematologic neoplasia: Some unusual manifestations. *Ann Intern Med 52:523–533.*

Shilkin, K. B., Annear, D. I., Rowett, L. R., and Laurence, B. H. (1968): Infection due to Aeromonas hydrophila. *Med J Aust 1:351–353.*

Sickles, E. A., Greene, W. H., and Wiernik, P. H. (1975): Clinical presentation of infection in granulocytopenic patients. *Arch Intern Med 135:715–719.*

Sickles, E. A., Young, V. M., Greene, W. H., and Wiernik, P. H. (1973): Pneumonia in acute leukemia. *Ann Intern Med 79:528–534.*

Siegel, S. E., Lunde, M. N., Gelderman, A. H., Halterman, R. H., Brown, J. A., Levine, A. S., and Graw, R. G., Jr. (1971): Transmission of toxoplasmosis by leukocyte transfusion. *Blood 37:383–394.*

Siguier, F., Godeau, P., Abelanet, R., De Saint-Maur, P., Nevot, P., and Sicard, D. (1970): Cryptococcose disséminée révélatrice d'un hépatome et d'un cancer du rein. *Ann Med Interne 121:523–530.*

Silver, R. T. (1963): Infections, fever and host resistance in neoplastic diseases. *J Chron Dis 16:677–701.*

Singer, C., Armstrong, D., Rosen, P. P., and Schottenfeld, D. (1975): *Pneumocystis carinii* pneumonia: a cluster of eleven cases. *Ann Intern Med 82:772–777.*

Sinkovics, J. G., and Smith, J. P. (1969): Salmonellosis complicating neoplastic diseases. *Cancer 24:631–636.*

Sinkovics, J. G., and Smith, J. P. (1970): Septicemia with bacteroides in patients with malignant disease. *Cancer 25:663–671.*

Slater, J. M., Ngo, E., and Lau, B. H. S. (1976): Effect of therapeutic irradiation on the immune response. *Am J. Roentgen Radium Ther Nucl Med 126:313–320.*

Smith, E., and Gaspar, I. A. (1968): Pentamidine treatment of pneumocystis carinii pneumonitis in an adult with lymphatic leukemia. *Am J Med 44:626–631.*

Smith, M. G. M., Golding, P. L., Eddleston, A. L. W. F., Mitchell, C. G., Kemp, A., and Williams, R. (1972): Cell-mediated immune responses in chronic liver diseases. *Br Med J 1:527–530.*

Smits, R. G., Krause, C. J., and Maccabe, B. F. (1972): Complications associated with combined therapy of oral and pharyngeal neoplasms. *Ann Otol Rhinol Laryngol 81:496–500.*

Smyth, D., Tripp, J. H., Brett, E. M., Marshall, W. C., Almeida, J., Dayan. A. D., Coleman, J. C., and Dayton, R. (1976): Atypical measles encephalitis in leukaemic children in remission. *Lancet 2:574.*

Sokal, J. E. (1966): Discussion on manifestations of immunological unresponsiveness in Hodgkin's disease. *Cancer Res 26:1161–1164.*

Sokal, J. E., Aungst, C. W., and Snyderman, M. (1974): Delay in progression of malignant lymphoma after BCG vaccination. *N Engl J Med 291:1226–1230.*

Sokal, J. E., and Firat, D. (1965): Varicella-zoster infection in Hodgkin's disease. *Am J Med 39:452–463.*

Sokal, J. E., and Shimaoka, K. (1967): Pyrogen in the urine of febrile patients with Hodgkin's disease. *Nature 215:1183–1185.*

Soussy, C. J., Squinazi, F. J., and Duval, J. (1975): Les Aeromonas en pathologie humaine. A propos de vingt observations personnelles. *Med Mal Infect 5:11–19.*

Southam, C. M., and Siegel, A. H. (1966): Serum levels of second components of complement in cancer patients. *J Immunol 97:331–337.*

Sparks, F. C., Silverstein, M. J., Hunt, J. S., Haskell, C. M., Pilch, Y. H., and Morton, D. L. (1973): Complications of BCG immunotherapy in patients with cancer. *N Engl J Med 289:827–830.*

Stevens D. A., Jordan, G. W., Wadell, T. F., and Merigan, T. C. (1973): Adverse effect of cytosine arabinoside on disseminated zoster in a controlled trial. *N Engl J Med 289:873–878.*

Steinberg, D., Gold, J., and Brodin, A. (1973): Necrotizing enterocolitis in leukemia. *Arch Intern Med 131:538–544.*

Steinberg, S. C., Halter, J. A., and Leventhal, B. G. (1975): The risk of hepatitis transmission to family contacts of leukemia patients. *J Pediat 87:753–756.*

Stumacher, R. J., Kovnat, M. J., and McCabe, W. R. (1973): Limitations of the usefulness of the limulus assay for endotoxin. *N Engl J Med 288:1261–1264.*

Suciu-Foca, N., Buda, J., McManus, J., Thiem, T., and Reemtsma, K. (1973): Impaired responsiveness of lymphocytes and serum inhibitory factors in patients with cancer. *Cancer Res 33:2373–2377.*

Sullivan, M. P., Hanshaw, J. B., Cangir, A., and Butler, J. J. (1968): Cytomegalovirus coplement-fixation antibody levels of leukemic children. Results of a longitudinal study. *J Am Med Assoc 206:569–574.*

Sullivan, P. W., and Salmon, S. E. (1972): Kinetics of growth and regression in IgG multiple myeloma. *J Clin Invest 51:1697–1708.*

Surgalla, M. J., Netter, E., and Fitzpatrick, J. (1975): Antibody response of patients with malignancies to bacteremia with gram-negative bacteria. *J Clin Microbiol 1:298–301.*

Sutherland, R. M., Inch, W. R., and McCredie, J. A. (1971): Phytohemagglutinin (PHA)-induced transformation of lymphocytes from patients with cancer. *Cancer 27:574–578.*

Sutnick, A. I., London, W. T., and Blumberg, B. S. (1971): Susceptibility to leukemia: immunologic factors in Down's syndrome. *J Natl Cancer Inst 47:923–933.*

Sutnick, A. I., London, W. T., Blumberg, B. S., Yankee, R. A., Gerstley, B. J. S., and Millman, I. (1970): Australia antigen (a hepatitis associated antigen) in leukemia. *J Natl Cancer Inst 44:1241–1249.*

Sutton, R. N. P., Darby, C. W., and Gumpel, S. M. (1971): Cytomegalovirus infection in childhood leukaemia. *Br J Haematol 20:437–442.*

Symposium (1973a): Optimal antimicrobial therapy in patients with cancer. *Eur J Cancer 9:393–458.*

Symposium (1973b): Herpes virus and cervical cancer. *Cancer Res 83:1345–1563.*

Symposium (1973c): Immunological aspects of Hodgkin's disease. *Tumori 59:341–388.*

Takita, H. (1970): Effect of postoperative empyema on survival of patients with bronchogenic carcinoma. *J Thorac Cardiovasc Surg* 59:642–644.

Tally, F. P., Lovie, T. J., Weinstein, W. M., Bartlett, J. G., and Gorbach, S. L. (1975): Amikacin therapy for severe gram negative sepsis. *Ann Intern Med* 83:484–488.

Tapper, M. L:, and Armstrong, D. (1974): Bacteremia due to *Pseudomonas* aeruginosa complicating neoplastic disease: a progress report. *J Infect Dis 130 (suppl.):* S14–S23.

Tapper, M. L., and Armstrong, D. (1976): Malaria complicating neoplastic disease. *Arch Intern Med 136:870–810.*

Tattersall, M. H. N., Hutchinson, R. M., Gaya, H., and Spiers, A. S. D. (1973): Empirical antibiotic therapy in febrile patients with neutropenia and malignant disease. *Eur J Cancer 9:417–423.*

Tattersall, M. H. N., Spiers, A. S. D., and Darrell, J. H. (1972): Initial therapy with combination of five antibiotics in febrile patients with leukemia and neutropenia. *Lancet 1:162–165.*

Tillotson, J. R., and Finland, M. (1969): Bacterial colonisation and clinical superinfection of the respiratory tract complicating antibiotic treatment of pneumonia. *J Infec Dis 119:597–624.*

Toala, P., Schroeder, S. A., Daly, A. K., and Finland, M. (1970): Candida at Boston City Hospital. Clinical and epidemiological characteristics and susceptibility to eight antimicrobial agents. *Arch Intern Med 126:983–989.*

Tobias, J. S., Brown, B. L., Brivkalns, A., and Yankee, R. A. (1976): Prophylactic granulocyte support in experimental septicemia. *Blood 47:473–479.*

Townsend, J. J., Wolinsky, J. S., Baringer, J. R., and Johnson, P. C. (1975): Acquired toxoplasmosis. A neglected cause of treatable nervous system disease. *Arch Neurol 32:335–343.*

Tuazon, C. V., and Sheagren, J. N. (1976): Teichoic acid antibodies in the diagnosis of serious infections with Staphylococcus aureus. *Ann Intern Med 84:543–546.*

Tugwell, P., and Greenwood, B. M. (1974): Bacteriological findings in pneumonia. *Lancet 1:95.*

Twomey, J. J. (1973): Infections complicating multiple myeloma and chronic lymphocytic leukemia. *Arch Intern Med 132:562–565.*

Utz, J. P., Garrigues, I. L., Sande, M. A., Warner, J. F., Mandell, G. L., McGehee, R. F., Duma, R. J., Shadomy, S. (1975): Therapy of cryptococcosis with a combination of flucytosine and amphotericin B. *J Infect Dis 132:368–373.*

Valdivieso, M., Luna, M., Bodey, G. P., Rodriguez, V., and Gröschel, D. (1976): Fungemia due to Torulopsis glabrata in the compromised host. *Cancer 38:1750–1756.*

Vallejos, C., McCredie, K. B., Bodey, G. P., Hester, J. P., and Freireich, E. J. (1975). White blood cell transfusions for control of infections in neutropenic patients. *Transfusion 15:28–33.*

Van Herik, M. (1965): Fever as a complication of radiation therapy for carcinoma of the cervix. *Am J Roentgenol Radium Ther Nucl Med 93:104–109.*

Vedder, J. A., and Scharr, W. F. (1969): Primary disseminated pulmonary aspergillosis with metastatic skin nodules. Successful treatment with inhalation nystatin therapy. *J. Am Med Assoc 209:1191–1195.*

Vich, Z. (1966): Beitrag zum Vorkommen van Herpes Zoster bei Patienten mit durch ionisierende Strahlen behandelten bösartigan Geschwülsten. *Strahlentherapie 130:198–204.*

Vietzke, W. M., Gelderman, A. H., Grimley, P. M., and Valsamis, M. P. (1968): Toxoplasmosis complicating malignancy. Experience at the National Cancer Institute. *Cancer 21:816–827.*

Vodopick, H., Chaskes, S. J., Solomon, A., and Stewart, J. A. (1947). Transient monoclonal gammopathy associated with cytomegalovirus infection. *Blood 44:189–195.*

Voisin, C., Goudemand, M., Wattel, F., Leduc, M., Bauters, F., Wallaert. C., and Beguery, P. (1970): Manifestations pleuro-pulmonaries au cours des leucémies. *J Fr Med Chir Thorac 24:505–521.*

Wagener, D. J. T., Van Munster, P. J. J., and Haanen, C. (1976): The immunoglobulins in Hodgkin's disease. *Eur J Cancer 12:683–688.*

Walzer, P. D., Perl, D. P., Krogstad, D. J., Rawson, P. G., and Schultz, M. G. (1974): *Pneumocystis carinii* pneumonia in the United States. Epidemiologic, diagnostic and clinical features. *Ann Intern Med 80:83–93.*

Ward, P. A., and Berenberg, J. L. (1974): Defectve regulation of inflammatory mediators in Hodgkin's disease. *N Engl J Med 290:76–80.*

Waterhouse, C. (1975): γ G-Globulin production and light-chain metabolism in patients with metastic cancer. *Cancer Res 35:987–990.*

Wegmann, T., Rohner, B., Müller, H. L. (1971): Die Candida-Serologie bei progredienten malignen Tumoren und Lungeninfekten. Ein Beitrag zur Diagnostik der Candidiasis. *Schweiz Med Wschr 101:1271–1274.*

Weiden, P. L., and Schuffler, M. D., (1974): Herpes esophagitis complicating Hodgkin's disease. *Cancer 33:1100–1102.*

Weiner, L. P., Johnson, R. T., and Herndon, R. M. (1973): Viral infections and demyelinating diseases. *N Engl J Med 288:1103–1110.*

Weinstein, L., Chang, T. W. (1973): The chemotherapy of viral infections. *N Engl J Med 289:725–730.*

Whittaker, K., Rees, K., and Clark, C. G. (1971): Reduced lymphocyte transformation in breast cancer. *Lancet 1:892–893.*

Whitecar, J. P., Jr., Luna M. and Bodey, G. P. (1970): Pseudomonas bacteremia in patients with malignant diseases. *Am J Med Sci 260:216–223.*

Whitley, R. J., Ch'ien, L. T., Dolin, R., Galasso, G. J., and Alford, C. A. (1976): Adenine arabinoside therapy of herpes-zoster in the immunodepressed. NIAID collaborative antiviral study. *N Engl J Med 294:1193–1199.*

Whittingham, S., Pitt, D. B., Sharma, D. L. B., and Mackay, I. R. (1977): Stress deficiency of the T-lymphocyte system exemplified by Down's syndrome. *Lancet 1:163–166.*

Whittle, H. C., Tugwell, C. P., Egler, L. J., and Greenwood, B. M. (1974): Rapid bacteriological diagnosis of pyrogenic meningitis by latex agglutination. *Lancet 2:619–621.*

Widholm, O., and Mattsson, T. (1972): Urinary tract infections in association with radium therapy for gynecological cancer. *Acta Obstet Gynecol Scand 51:247–250.*

Wiernick, P. H., and Serpick, A. A. (1969): Pulmonary embolus in acute myelocytic leukemia. *Cancer 24:581–584.*

Wilkinson, P. M., Sumner, C., Delamore, I. W., Geary, C. G., and Milner, G. R. (1975): Granulocyte function in myeloblastic leukaemia. *Br J Cancer 32:574–577.*

Williams, H. M., Diamond, H. D., Craver, L. F., Parsons, H. (1959): *Neurological Complications of Lymphomas and Leukemias.* Thomas, Springfield, Ill.

Wilson, B. D., Surgalla, M. J., and Yates, J. W. (1974): Aerobic and anaerobic surgical wound contamination in patients with cancer. *Surg Gynecol Obstet* 139:329–332.

Wolf, P., Dorfman, R., and McClenahan, J. (1970): False-positive infectious mononucleosis spot test in lymphoma. *Cancer 25:626–628.*

Wolfe, M. S., Armstrong, D., Louria, D. B., and Blevins, A. (1971): Salmonellosis in patients with neoplastic disease. *Arch Intern Med 128:546–554.*

Wolff, S. M., Dale, D. C., Clark, R. A., Root, R. K., and Kimball, H. R. (1972): Chediak-Higashi syndrome: studies of host defenses. *Ann Intern Med 76:293–306.*

Wolstenholme, G. E. W., and Birch, J. (1971): *Pyrogens and Fever.* Livingstone, London.

Worms, P. (1969): Etat actuel des septicémies à staphylocoques. *Rev Prat Paris 19:1945–1959.*

Wright, E. T., and Winer, L. H. (1961): Herpes zoster and malignancy. *Arch Derm Chicago 84:242–244.*

Wuttke, A. (1974): Lymphogranulomatose mit Toxoplasmose-Enzephalitis. *Dtsch Med Wschr 99:1689–1691.*

Wynne, J. W., and Armstrong, D. (1972): Clostridial septicemia. *Cancer 29:215–221.*

Yates, J. W., and Holland, J. F. (1973): A controlled study of isolation and endogenous microbial suppression in acute myelocytic leukemia patients. *Cancer 32:1490–1498.*

Yim, Y., Kikkawa, Y., Tanowitz, H., and Wittner, M. (1970): Fatal strongyloîdiasis in Hodgkin's disease after immunosuppressive therapy. *J Trop Med Hyg 10:245–249.*

Young, C. W., and Dowling, M. D., Jr. (1975): Antipyretic effect of cycloheximide, an inhibitor of protein synthesis, in patients with Hodgkin's disease or other malignant neoplasms. *Cancer Res 35:1218–1224.*

Young, L. S., Armstrong, D., Blevins, A., and Lieberman, P. (1971): Nocardia asteroîdes infection complicating neoplastic disease. *Am J Med 50:356–367.*

Young, L. S., Meyer, R. D., and Armstrong, D. (1973): Controlled prospective trial of *Pseudomonas aeruginosa* vaccine in cancer patients. *Ann Intern Med 79:518–527.*

Young, R. C. (1969): The Budd-Chiari syndrome caused by *Aspergillus.* Two patients with vascular invasion of the hepatic veins. *Arch Intern Med 124:754–757.*

Young, R. C., Bennett, J. E. (1971): Invasive aspergillosis. Absence of detectable antibody response. *Am Rev Resp Dis 104:710–716.*

Young, R. C., Bennett, J. E., Vogel, C. L., Carbone, P. P., and DeVita, V. T. (1970): Aspergillosis: the spectrum of the disease in 98 patients. *Medicine 49:147–173.*

Zimmermann, L. E. (1955): Fatal fungus infections complicating other diseases. *Am J Clin Pathol 25:46–65.*

Zornoza, J., Goldman, A. M., Wallace, S., Valdivieso, M., and Bodey, G. P. (1976): Radiologic features of Gram-negative pneumonias in the neutropenic patient. *Am J Roentgenol Radium Ther Nucl Med 127:989–996.*

ZuRhein, G. M., and Chou, S. M. (1965): Particles resembling papova viruses in human cerebral demyelinating disease. *Science 148:1477–1479.*

# Index

Adenine-arabinoside, 98, 149
*Aeromonas*, 77–79
Agammaglobulinemia, 17
Alcohol, 18, 133
Amantadine, 98
Amikacin, 142
Aminoglycosides, 143, 149
Aminosides, 142, 143, 145
Amphotericin B, 105, 109, 112, 113, 114, 115, 137, 148
Ampicillin, 137, 143–147
Anaerobic agents, 65, 73, 84
Anemia, 39
Anguillulosis, 13
Antibiotics, 28, 57, 140–150, 155, 156
    prophylactic therapy, 136–138
    resistance to, 66
Antibodies, 60
Anticancer treatment, 23–28, 129–132, 161
Antigen, 61
Antigen–antibody reaction, 60
Anti-infectious treatment, 132–139, 140–150
Asparaginase, 41
Aspergillosis, 61, 109–112
*Aspergillus*, 6, 14, 15, 104, 109–112
Ataxia-telangiectasia, 16

*Bacilli*, 83
*Also see* Gram-negative bacilli
Bacterial infections, 5–7, 42, 55, 65–89, 157, 159
*Bacteroides*, 12, 84–85
Barriers, 155
BCG, 87
    test, 23, 134
Beta-lactamines, 142, 143, 145
Biological diagnosis, 53–61

Biopsies, 23
Blastomycosis, 104, 115
Bleomycin, 41
Blood, cultures, 57
    fractions, 150–153
    malignant disease, 49–52, 89, 94
Bovine tuberculosis bacillus, 87
Breast cancer, 82, 86
Bronchopulmonary infections, 66–70
Burkitt's lymphoma, 90, 91

Cancer, infections in, 3–15, 154–155, 157–159
    patient–cancer–infection relationship, 32–37
    and viruses, 90–91
*Candida*, 6, 8, 14, 31, 58, 103–105, 106–109
Candidiasis, 49, 61, 104, 105, 106–109
    esophageal, 12
Carbenicillin, 142–147, 149
Catheters, 28, 45
Cell-mediated immunity, 20–21
Cephalosporins, 143, 149
Cephalothin, 142–147
Chediak-Higashi disease, 17
Chemotherapy, 26–27, 33, 41, 87, 92, 93–94, 155, 160
    anti-infectious, 140–150
Children, 96
Cholestasis, 48
Chromoblastosis, 104, 115
Cleaning act, 130
Clinical diagnosis, 42–52
*Clostridium*, 83–85
Clotrimazole, 105
*Coccidioides*, 103, 105
Coccidioidomycosis, 115
Colonization, 30

193

Coma, 118
Complement, 22
Congenital conditions, 16–17
Contamination, 31–32
Corticosteroids, 98, 132
*Corynebacterium equi*, 83
Cotrimoxazole, 120, 124
Counterimmunoelectrophoresis, 59, 60
Cryptococcosis, 113–114
*Cryptococcus*, 6, 104, 105
Cryptogenic abnormalities, 17–18
Curative treatment, 140–153
Cutaneous manifestation of infection, 14, 48
Cyanosis, 122
Cycloserine, 88
Cytarabine, 41, 98
*Cytomegalovirus*, 6, 7, 60, 100

Death, 157–159
Dental care, 133
Diagnosis of infections, 3–4, 42–61
    biologic, 53–61
    clinical, 42–52
    early, 161
    laboratory, 54
Diarrhea, 48
Digestive manifestation of infection, 48
Direct investigation, 55–59
DNA autosomes, 66
Down's syndrome, 17
Dysenteric syndrome, 48
Dysglobulinemia, 72
Dysphagia, 49
Dyspnea, 67

Ecology, microbial, 15
Elderly patients, 18
Emetine, 98
Empyema, 154
Encephalitis, 118
Encephalopathy, 102
Endobronchial brush biopsy, 124
Endoscopies, 23
*Enterobacter*, 15, 66
*Enterobacteriaceae*, 30, 65
Entry, portal of, 45, 52, 58
Eosinophilia, 53, 126
Epidemiology of cancer infection, 3–15, 16

Epstein–Barr virus, 90–92
Erythema, 117
*Escherichia coli*, 66, 68, 75, 142, 158
Ethambutol, 88

Fever, 13, 37–41, 67, 140–141, 149, 159
    in diagnosis, 43–45
    in parasitic infections, 117
    in septicemia, 52
Flora, 29, 137
Flu, 101–102
Flucytosine, 105, 112, 113, 114, 148
Fungal infections, 8, 103–115, 148, 157–158, 160
Fungi, 65, 101
*Fusobacterium necrophorum*, 85

Gallium-citrate scanning, 58
Gamma globulins, 98, 135, 153
Gastrointestinal cancers, 81, 82, 84
Gentamicin, 137, 142–147, 150–151
Geotrichosis, 115
*Geotrichum*, 104
Gram-negative bacilli, 60, 65–66, 68, 75, 81, 157, 160
Gram-positive bacilli, 65
Gram-positive cocci, 65, 80
Granulocytopenia, 43, 44, 49–52, 53, 65, 67–69, 70, 75, 149
Granulocytosis, 132

Hb antigen, 90–92
*Haemophilus aphrophilus*, 79
HeLa cells, 100
Hematology, 3
    malignancies, 7
Hepatic manifestation of infection, 48
Hepatitis, 48, 92
    viral, 102
Herpes virus, 3, 7, 24
    *hominis*, 99
    simplex type-2, 90, 92
    zoster, 92–98, 135, 156, 159
*Histoplasma*, 104
Histoplasmosis, 114
Hodgkin's disease, 3, 7, 9, 11, 14, 20, 34, 69, 76, 85–86, 91, 93, 95, 110, 117, 118–119, 121, 125, 131, 154, 156
Hospitalism, 14–15, 30

Hospitalization, 57
hygiene, 133
Humoral immunity, 20
Hygiene, 18, 133, 139

Idoxurudine, 98, 148
Immunity, 20–21
Immunsofluorescence test, 61
Immunoglobulins, 16, 98, 135, 150, 153
Immunologic deficiencies, 16, 17, 131
Immunoprophylaxis, 134–136
Immunosuppression, 20, 35, 61, 155
Immunotherapy, 27–28
Infections, 42–43
    and cancer, 3–15, 154–155, 157
    epidemiology, 3–15
    factors favoring, 16–28
    lethal, 157–159
    localized, 45
    viral, 12, 90–102
Infectious fevers, 39
Interferon, 22
Investigations, 23
Iritis, 94
Irradiation, 13–14, 23–24, 25, 150, 159
    and fever, 41
    and herpetic infection, 100
Isolation, 138, 161
Isoniazide, 88

Jaundice, 48

Kanamycin, 144–147
Keratitis, 94
Klebsiella, 66, 68, 75, 143, 158
Klebsiella-Enterobacter, 15
Koch's bacillus, 101

Laboratory diagnosis, 54
Latex-particle agglutination, 59
Lesions, 51, 129–131
Lethal infections, 157–159
Leukemia, 7, 9, 14, 15, 21, 34–36, 49,
    74, 76, 81, 82, 84, 110, 125, 149,
    158
    acute, 138–139
    and bacterial infections, 65, 70, 72
    and candidiasis, 106–107
    chronic lymphoid, 132

and herpes virus, 92, 95
and leukocytes, 151–152
and parasitic infection, 117, 121
and varicella, 96
Leukocytes, 151–153, 161
    functions, 22
    leukocytic concentrates, 139
Leukoencephalopathy, 102
Leukopenia, 21
*Limulus* test, 53
*Listeria*, 6
    *monocytogenes*, 82
Lung cancer, 82, 85–87
Lymphadenitis, 87
Lymphadenopathy, 119
Lymphangiography, 39–41
Lymph-node manifestations of infection,
    48
Lymphomas, 34, 36, 72, 74, 76, 81–82,
    84, 87, 110, 125
    Burkitt's, 90, 91
    malignant, 11, 85
    and parasitic infections, 117, 121

Maduromycosis, 104
Malaria, 126
Malnutrition, 11, 13
Measles, 101, 134
Medical intervention, 22–28
Medications, 28
Melanoma, 7
Meningitis, 72, 74, 107
    cryptococcal, 113
    meningeal manifestations of infection,
    49
Meningo-encephalitis, 94, 107
Microbial contamination, 29–31
Microorganisms, 29–31, 65–89
*Also see* Bacteria
Mononucleosis, 101
*Mucor,* 6
Mucorales, 104, 114
Mucormyosis, 114
Mycobacterial infections, 85–89, 158
Mycobacteriosis, 88–89
*Mycoplasma pneumoniae,* 69–70
Mycoplasmas, 12
Mycosis, 12, 155
    fungoides, 9
Myelomas, 34, 35–36, 74

NBT dye test, 53
Necrotizing pneumopathy, 51
Neomycin B, 137
Neoplasms, 42
Neoplastic ulceration, 19
Neurologic manifestation of infection, 14
Neutropenia, 132
Neutrophil migration, 22
*Nocardia asteroides,* 69
Nonspecific reactions, 21–22
Nystatin, 105, 109, 137, 148

Obligate anaerobic agents, 65, 73, 83–85
Obstruction, 65
Oncology, 136, 138, 162
Orientation tests, 53–55

Paraneoplastic fevers, 37–39
Paraneoplastic immune deficiency, 93, 129–132
Parasarcoidosis, 91
Parasitic infections, 9, 12, 116–126, 159
Parasitosis, 125
Pathology, interlocking, 155–157
Pathophysiology, 29–41
Patient–cancer–infection relationship, 32–37
Perianal abcesses, 70–72
Perirectal abcesses, 70–72
Phagocytosis, 21, 49
*Phycomycetes,* 104
Plasmids, 66
Pleuropulmonary manifestations of infection, 46–47
*Pneumococcus,* 15, 46, 80, 82, 158
*Pneumocystis carinii,* 101
Pneumocystosis, 9, 10, 12–13, 14, 61, 116, 120–125, 160
Pneumonia, 12, 14, 69, 94, 118
   bacterial, 67
   interstitial, 51, 58–59
Polymyxin, 142
Polypeptides, 142
Portal of entry, 45, 52, 58
Potassium iodide, 114
Preventive treatment, 129–139
Prognosis, 159
Prophylactic antibiotic therapy, 136–138
*Proteus,* 66, 68, 142, 143, 158
*Pseudomonas,* 6, 12, 14, 15, 30, 31–32,

66, 68, 75–77, 78, 143, 158
   and aspergillosis, 110
   and vaccination, 134–135
Pulmonary manifestation of infections, 14, 46–47, 51
Pyrimethanin, 120
Pyrogens, 37, 38, 39

Radiotherapy, 23–24, 93–94, 131
Reactions (nonspecific), 21–22
R factor, 66
Rhodorula, 115
Rifampicin, 88, 142
RTF (resistance transfer factor), 66
Rubella, 156
   *Also see* Measles

*Salmonella,* 77
Salmonellosis, 5, 77
Sanitation, 132–133
Schistosomiasis, 126
Septicemias, 12, 52–53, 55, 67–69, 72–85, 148
   and candidiasis, 107
   and leukocytes, 151
Serologic tests, 59–61, 119
*Serratia,* 66, 77
Smallpox, 134
Smoking, 18, 133
Spiramycin, 120
Splenectomy, 26
Splenomegaly, 52
Sporotrichosis, 104
Staphylococcemia, 60
*Staphylococcus,* 80, 143, 158
   vaccination, 135
Stenosis, 65
Strongyloides, 125–126
Sulfamethoxazole, 124, 145
Sulfonamides, 120
Superinfections, 18, 46, 91–92, 129
Surgery, 24–26, 150
Systemic abnormalities, 16–18

Tests, serologic, 59–61
Thiabendazole, 126
Thrombocytopenia, 94
Thromboembolism, 42
Ticarcillin, 142, 143–147, 149
Titers, 60

*Torulopsis,* 103, 104, 115
  *glabrata,* 8
*Toxoplasma,* 6
Toxoplasmosis, 61, 116–120
Transfer factor, 132
Transfusion, 28
Trimethoprim, 124
Tuberculosis, 5–7, 85–87, 88
Tubramycin, 144–147
Tumor, 33–35, 42, 76, 117, 121, 130, 158
  compressive, 124
  favoring infections, 18–22

Ulceration, 19, 65, 110

Urogenital cancer, 81

Vaccines, 134–136
Vancomycin, 137
Varicella, 92–98, 135
Viral infections, 12, 90–102, 157–158
Viruses, 90–91

Weil-Fely reactions, 61
Wiskott-Aldrich syndrome, 17

*Yersinia enterocolitica,* 79

X-Rays, 122